To my friend Tom,

Reversing Chronic Disease

Other Books by the same author:

Beating Alzheimer's, Penguin Putnam, East Rutherford, NJ, 1989.

Reversing Chronic Disease

Getting Well Again

Tom Warren

Capital University School of Integrated Medicine, Washington, D.C.

Published by:

New Century Press
1055 Bay Blvd., Suite C
Chula Vista, CA 91911
800-519-2465
www.newcenturypress.com

Tom Warren's web page: www.beatingchronicdisease.com

ISBN catalog number: 1-890035-22-X

Book design by Michèle Savelle
University of Washington, Seattle, WA
Cover design by David W. Ehlert, MAMS, CMI
University of Washington, Seattle, WA

Printed with non-toxic ink.

Printed in the United States of America.

Table of Contents

Section Two - For Medical Professionals

Appendix VI

Appendix VII

Appendix VIII

Appendix IX

Appendix X

Appendix XI

Appendix XII

Appendix XIII

Appendix XIV-1

Appendix XIV-2

Foreword

"It requires a very unusual mind to undertake the analysis of the obvious." — *Alfred North Whitehead*

Whatever your philosophical conviction, it is a fact that Man has been endowed with a genetic code of the built-in information for natural survival. However, the data stored in the chemical bonds of our DNA are apparently designed to handle environmental change (slowly). While Man lived in hunter-gathering tribal groups, forging subsistence from a competitive and dangerous world, change was relatively slow. Today however, Man has divorced himself from his biological roots, preferring to live in complex artificial electronic castles, safe from the forces of natural variation. True, we still breathe the air, drink the water and feast on the cornucopia of plant life. But more often than not, the air is polluted with noxious chemicals of industry, the water "fortified" with chlorine and fluoride and pesticides residues permeates our genetically modified and low-level irradiated sterilized foods. It is a fact! We are too smart for our own good.

The "rub" is that our own health care providers have bought into "progress," without stopping to examine their procedures with common sense. Blinded by the medical paradigm, the dental profession is no exception, choosing to medicate the mouths of children with a timed-released poison. A poison that Hippocrates, the Father of Medicine, warned about centuries ago: a poison called mercury. Mercury found in your "silver" fillings!

Blinded by the medical paradigm, the dental profession has chosen to retain dead teeth through root canal treatment, leaving bacteria behind to grow and mutate in a location inaccessible to the human immune system. Leaving bacteria behind to produce toxins that diffuse from the protected innards of the tooth into systemic circulation. If that is not bad enough, dead remnants of your own tissue remain in the over three miles of tubules in the tooth's dentine layer. Tissue remnants that putrefy and become gangrenous may not exhibit overt symptoms for decades.

Blinded by the medical paradigm, the dental profession has chosen to recommend "fortification" of our drinking water—mass medicating every man woman or child with the promise of no cavities. If cavities were caused by fluoride deficiency, maybe a case could be made. However, tooth decay is a nutritional disease of refined sugar consumption. It is like chasing a headache with pain medication. You are never sure what is causing the headache, are you?

Blinded by the medical paradigm, the dental profession refers you to the dental hygienist, to scrap and scratch your infected gums, causing bacteria to be forced into your blood stream, putting you at risk to serious general infection.

These are only a few of the many atrocities perpetrated by an unthinking profession. Trapped in their paradigm, dentists don't see the forest for the trees. Yet often individuals, within and outside a professional group, lift their heads up to try to smell fresh air. Tom Warren is one such person. And, this book addresses many important health issues. Tom raises many questions and answers quite a few. To the best of his ability he melds personal enthusiasm, case histories and science. Tom Warren is an "unusual mind." And this is an unusually useful book.

Thanks, Tom.

Murray J. Vimy, D.M.D.,Dentist
Clinical Associate Professor of Medicine
University of Calgary, Canada

Old Tom– New Tom

When I think back to that day in 1984 when I first met Tom Warren, and compare it with our conversations in 2002, it is gratifying that I cannot connect the two Toms as being the same person. If anyone has shown that Alzheimer's disease is not a downhill slide, it is Tom Warren.

From a wandering body with a confused, dazed mind, to a fighter with design and purpose for those who wander down the path of eventual self-destruction, Tom has given us all reason to continue to press forward. He is not fighting for his own life like he was when I first met him. He is now dedicated to abolishing that path so others do not have to face the tigers he faced — and defeated.

His energy gains momentum each year, although there is no yardstick to measure it. Tom doesn't have milestones and rewards to encourage him on. He just lifts his pen as if it were a machete and clears away the tangled vines of science that hinder progress. Thank you, New Tom, for being our torchbearer.

Hal Huggins, D.D.S., M.S.

Tom Warren continues to amaze. His first major writing effort, *Beating Alzheimer's*, was especially impressive. Not only did Tom describe his own decline in mental function because of dental toxicity, he also showed that his recovery was complete enough to allow a detailed and accurate description of his fighting experience. Furthermore, information offered in his first book was all the more impressive in light of Tom's absence of formal medical training. Doctors and the lay public alike can only benefit by reading about Tom's ordeal with minds as open as possible.

In this book, *Reversing Chronic Disease*, Tom Warren again writes with clarity and precision with a brain that he literally reclaimed from a disease that robs so many people of their dignity. Tom has impressively researched mountains of scientific data and once again produced a result that can benefit all who read it. Multiple case histories from victims of dental toxicity are included. The effects of dental toxicity are well addressed from medical, political, legal and emotional perspectives.

Tom, keep up the good work. You are an inspiration to us all.

Thomas Levy, M.D., J.D.

Reversing Chronic Disease is a critically important book.

If it were written by an Integrative Heath Professional, involved with the issues that Tom Warren so skillfully exposes, it would be discounted as fictional at worse and exaggerated at best.

The evidence is overwhelming that chronic low-level mercurial poisoning, other heavy metals and environmental pollution are causal, or at the very least a contributory factor involved with the chronic disease process. This book is clearly written and accurately documents the facts for the patient and professional to understand.

Thank you Tom, I believe every patient who is not being helped by conventional therapy should read *Reversing Chronic Disease*.

Mark J. McClure, D.D.S.
Doctor of Integrative Medicine
Provost - Capital University of Integrative Medicine
Professor - Department of Applied Neurobiology

Disclaimer

Everyone is unique. I cannot personally see those who suffer from Alzheimer's, control their environment or know if they are physically and mentally healthy enough or have the motivation to travel the path that I took to reverse the condition neurologists call Alzheimer's disease. Therefore, the following disclaimer is legally necessary.

This information is for educational purposes only. As with any information that could affect your health, the author and the publisher encourage the reader to discuss the details herein with his or her health care provider. I am not a medical professional and I cannot promise that if the Alzheimer's sufferer does everything possible to follow the treatment protocol herein, he or she will recover. The fact that other people have regained their health and short-term memory does not guarantee everyone will be so fortunate.

Dedication

To Jesus Christ: After I was diagnosed with Alzheimer's disease, I cried out "Lord save me!" That was over twenty years ago, and today I am alive because of Him. The Lord did not save me because I was a good man. I wasn't. I think He saved me because I asked, "Jesus, if I have to die this death, at least through me let the cure for Alzheimer's disease be found." I take no credit for this book. None.

To my wife, Louise, who loved and supported me, and without whose help I would have died years ago.

To my children, who suffered the slings and arrows of my explosive, twisted thought process. They paid a higher price than I. If it were not for the opportunity to write *Beating Alzheimer's Disease* and this book, *Reversing Chronic Disease*, I would have preferred to die before causing our family to suffer so much devastation and heartache. Mental illness destroys every vestige of normal family life.

Acknowledgements

Looking back over two decades, I met some of the finest men and women in the world: physicians, dentists, researchers, writers, attorneys, caregivers and friends who suffered from all sorts of chronic diseases who have recovered their health after removing their mercury amalgam fillings and root canals. The price they paid to get this message to the public is inconceivable. If there are any heroes in this book, it is those individuals.

When *Beating Alzheimer's* was first published in November of 1989, we were fighting some of the wealthiest, most powerful industries and medical specialties in the world. The United States, Canada, Sweden, Germany and other governments were involved in the cover-up of the amalgam issue because of economic reverberations. Hundreds of thousands of careers are threatened. Some men would rather die than publicly lose their self-esteem, their income and become virtual outcasts within their communities. That is the reason change evolves so slowly in medicine. Do not expect the medical establishment to admit that they allowed dentists to poison at least 80 percent of the American population. For those who know, the only thing I want to ask is: How can you live with yourselves?

Thanks to the Well Mind Association of Seattle, Washington, who put the books in my hand that saved my life, to DAMS (Dental Amalgam Mercury Syndrome group), and to Dr. Hal Huggins,[1] Dr. Murray

1 Dr. Sandra Denton insisted that I come down to Hal Huggins' dental clinic at Colorado Springs before she moved to Alaska. Thank God she did. I told Sandy that I did not have the money. I'd been ill a long time by then. Dr. Denton told me to work it out with Hal. So I called, explaining that I could pay only $400 a month, and Hal said, "Come on down." When I checked in I gave Hal's secretary a check for $400. The next day she asked me for a check for $265, which I gave her. Then she returned the $400 check. Hal is that way. I do not know how much the bill for cleaning out 20 jawbone infections should have cost fifteen years ago. In 2002 it would be more than $7,000.

Vimy, Dr. Roger Eichman, Dr. George Meinig, Dr. Patrick Störtebecker, Dr. Mats Hansen, Dr. John Ely, Dr. Horst Poehlmann, and Dr. Theron Randolph. Then there is author Sam Ziff, and his son Dr. Michael Ziff, Dr. Sandra Denton, Dr. Thomas Levy, Dr. Boyd Haley, Dr. Curt Pendergrass, Dr. Jerry Bouquot and Dr. Fritz Lorscheider. There are so many former mercury-toxic patients to whom I owe a thank you that it is impossible to remember all their names. John Moore and Murlene Brake ought to have their names among these heroes. They are two of the most selfless people I have ever known.

It would have been impossible to publish this work without Elaine Stannard, of the Seattle Well Mind Association, who made many thoughtful suggestions. Thanks to Carolyn Reeder for formatting this book through many revisions. Thank you to Sandra Duffy, a friend and an attorney who further edited this work. Dr. Andrew Cutler, PhD, and Dr. Allen Rowberg have been very helpful. Ed Baker, a retired editor for the Seattle Times, rounds out the editing group.

Charlie Brown, former Attorney General of the state of West Virginia and former staff attorney with the Federal Trade Commission, is the attorney spearheading litigation against the American Dental Association (ADA). Charlie told a group of us he was having a conversation with Dr. Huggins about dental amalgam issues and Dr. Huggins said, "Where else can you save a billion lives?" Charlie never looked back. He is currently involved in the Consumers for Dental Choice project, which is concerned with freedom of speech for dentists and freedom of information for dental patients. Thank you, Charlie.

Thank you all.

Chapter 1

Iatrogenic Disease – Misplaced Trust

Iatrogenic disease is disease caused by inappropriate medical treatment. Eventually everyone will die. But people shouldn't have to endure years of unnecessary suffering before they expire while paying medical expenses that impoverish the decedent's family. What if it was possible to be healthy, produce income, enjoy an active lifestyle and be mentally alert into the late 80's, perhaps longer? I tell shaggy-dog stories to many fellows with white hair. They burst out laughing and usually tell me, thanks, I made their day, or some similar comment. One fellow said, "Let's face it, there is no one older than me." Another said, "I am a hundred." Their thought processes were as clear as mine, and I'm seventy-one.

On the other side of the coin, I have talked with many young people who appear to be chronically ill. They are lethargic, unproductive workers. They are not enthusiastically in touch with their surroundings. Intuitively, they are vaguely aware something is not right. The way I put it to my doctor, an internist, before I was diagnosed with Alzheimer's disease was, "Can you be sick and not know it?" He gave me every test he could think of but found nothing wrong.

The symptoms of chronic low-level mercurial poisoning[2] are subtle and difficult to identify. And that's too bad, because the missing di-

2 Mercury can be deadly. Karen Wetterhahn, PhD, a usually careful scientist at Dartmouth, died after exposure to one drop of mercury.
(See appendix VII for the complete report.)

agnosis, the root cause of Alzheimer's disease and schizophrenia, is mercury toxicity. Once medical practitioners learn to recognize the subtle subclinical signs of chronic low-level mercurial poisoning, they will have identified the primary cause of Alzheimer's, autism, endogenous depression and schizophrenia. All of these conditions have similar subclinical symptoms.[3]

What About Other Diseases?

The identical procedures that reverse Alzheimer's also reverse many chronic diseases. Keep reading—see if the shoe fits. Twenty years ago I would have given everything we owned for the following information.

The Tip of the Iceberg

The Alzheimer's Association estimates there are approximately 37 million people suffering severe, deteriorating, short-term memory loss throughout the world. More than five million live in North America. Neurologists continually tell the whole world that Alzheimer's patients have an incurable disease. Fortunately, current medical dogma about the primary cause and cure for Alzheimer's disease is inaccurate. Provided the Alzheimer's sufferer can carry on a halfway reasonable conversation for five minutes, it is possible to recover. It's not easy. It takes work. It does cost money and most of all it takes knowledge, which is the purpose of this book.

As early as 1929, a Rio de Janeiro dentist, Dr. Olympio Pinto's father, reversed more "so called" incurable diseases than will be discussed herein by replacing silver fillings with high-quality gold. The term "silver filling" is a misnomer. The proper scientific name for any amalgam compound is its highest metal content. The correct scientific name for a silver amalgam dental filling is mercury amalgam dental filling.

---

3 See Appendix I.

Mercury dental fillings contain 50% mercury, 35% silver, 9% tin, 6% copper and a trace amount of zinc. Other metals, even zinc, synergistically potentiate mercury toxicity.

Divergent Interests

On one hand, our physicians and dentists are dedicated, caring professionals who do everything in their power to help their patients recover. Few of us would be willing to pay the price they do to put MD or DDS behind their name. The vast majority of these men and women deserve our admiration and respect. Notwithstanding, there are serious ethical and mounting legal problems within the dental community concerning the use of mercury amalgam dental fillings. A surprising number of ADA dentists and their spouses, when they know that they will not be quoted, are troubled and far more candid and pointed about the ADA's position on the mercury-amalgam issue than anything that I am willing to write.

In 1987 the ADA changed its code of ethics indicating mercury-amalgam fillings could be removed for cosmetic reasons, but the removal of mercury amalgam for health reasons was unethical and unprofessional conduct. If dentists informed their patients that 50% of a silver filling is mercury, a highly neurotoxic poison, the ADA arranged to have their dental licenses revoked by State Dental Boards. That is direct proof of a cover-up any jury can understand.

In Canada, representatives of the Canadian Dental Association went to the dean of the medical school at the University of Calgary to stop further research by the neuroscience team that first exposed mercury's toxicity to the North American medical community. They were unsuccessful.

The California Legislature voted 70 to 1 to disband their entire dental board as of December 31, 2001. When Governor Gray Davis fired all of them, he said the dental board was working for the ADA, not in the interests of dental patients.

It gives me no satisfaction to have written *Beating Alzheimer's* more than 13 years ago knowing that the root cause of Alzheimer's disease is iatrogenic disease while our population continued to be poisoned and the ADA stone-walled their culpability on the issue. During this time a minimum of 12 percent, or 960,000 of our population's immune systems, have been seriously damaged by mercury poisoning and have developed chronic diseases ranging from allergies and chemical sensitivities to cancer, type II diabetes, endogenous depression, schizophrenia, dementia, multiple sclerosis, amyotrophic lateral sclerosis, Parkinson's, Alzheimer's and dozens of other chronic diseases the traditional medical community has little understanding of and no cure for.

All the ballyhoo in television ads about dentistry is like looking at a one-eyed Jack. The public is not allowed to see the opposite face, the iatrogenic diseases mercury causes—any more than cigarette advertisements[4] would present a lung cancer patient lying on his deathbed. The ADA has repeated its lies about mercury for so long that even most of the medical community believes them. You will not find dental research extolling the virtues of mercury-amalgam in peer-review medical journals such as *FASEB, the AMA Journal, Lancet, or NeuroToxicology*. Their editors know better. Ask your dentist to show you one research paper proving mercury is safe for human tissue. If none exist, why would people put the stuff in their mouth? More importantly, why would parents allow the dentist to poison their children? "It's a bizarre conversation we're having here. The ADA is trying to argue that a poison is not a poison."[5]

The most accurate thing I can tell the reader is that there is continual conflict of interest by those who produce and sell hazardous products

---

4 September 23, 1999, the government filed a massive lawsuit against the tobacco industry to recover smoking-related health costs and immediately stood accused of hypocrisy for filing suit after colluding with the industry for decades.

5 Dr. Alfred P. Zamm, Environmental Medicine, UPO Box 4350, Kingston, NY 12402, M.W.F. 1PM to 8PM (914) 338-7766.

to the public and the people they have injured. Few businessmen intentionally produce or sell unsafe products. They usually learn of the problem later. Profit potential and fear of litigation cloud management's perspective. The sad thing is that the millions of people whose health has been destroyed will lose or have lost their earning capacity. Injured, sick, unemployed workers cannot afford to hire lawyers, lobbyists and public relations firms to look after and protect their interest. We expect our government to protect the public interest. Unfortunately, campaign financing inappropriately influences public policy. At the present time, until more of the American public becomes aware of the following information, politicians are not going to take action. It's not a level playing field and those of us whom our dentists injured have been written off. That's just the way it is, and that is the reason I continually tell those suffering from chronic low-level mercury poisoning from mercury amalgam dental fillings to take charge of your own recovery program. Most people can recover.

To reiterate: the same procedures that reverse Alzheimer's disease will also reverse schizophrenia and many other chronic diseases. As you treat each of the underlying symptoms, short-term memory loss fades into the background and remains a minor nuisance reminding you to continue to take care of your health.

The Cause

The primary source of Alzheimer's disease is inappropriate dental treatment that causes a whole host of related symptoms, e.g., food allergy, chemical sensitivities, destruction of brain tissue, arteriosclerosis, low stomach acid, candida overgrowth and leaky-gut syndrome, etc., that synergistically produce short-term memory loss. It does not matter if you have had false teeth for decades; you still have infection and mercury residues from old dental fillings in your body tissues. Mercury and waste products from anaerobic bacteria within jawbone infections and root canals poison you. In addition, lead, copper, and—

some studies suggest—aluminum[6] might have a toxic effect on brain tissue. Brain injury, alcoholism, arteriosclerosis, excitotoxins,[7] food allergy, leaky-gut syndrome, chemical sensitivity, candida overgrowth, mold, specific viruses and diabetes accelerate the disease process.

Some of the most toxic poisons in existence originate from jawbone infections and root canals. If dental patients really understood the pathology of jawbone infection, if this were 140 years ago, frontier cowboys would have tarred and feathered any itinerant quack who suggested doing a root canal. Get a bridge or a partial plate, but never, ever get a root canal. Root canals are akin to jumping out of an airplane without a parachute and the fellow you'll meet on the way down will be Digby O'Dell—the friendly undertaker. It gets worse; the pathologist won't even have a clue to the underlying cause of your demise. It will appear that you died from cancer, a heart attack, from diabetes or dozens of other chronic diseases. (Root canals will be covered in more detail in Chapter 2.)

Medical Politics

When the first edition of *Beating Alzheimer's* was published in November of 1989, I assumed doctors really wanted to know how to reverse the Alzheimer's disease process. Instead the medical community closed ranks and did their utmost to prevent the public from learning the primary cause of short-term memory loss and literally ran the dentists and physicians who knew the most about reversing Alzheimer's disease out of business, e.g., Dr. Hal Huggins' license to practice dentistry was revoked because he told the world that mer-

6 Many medicines contain aluminum. Antacids contain from44mg to 400mg per dose. Over-the-counter buffered aspirin contain up to 44mg. Over-the-counter anti-diarrhea drugs contain up to 600mg per tablet. Louis Blank, who recovered from Alzheimer's disease (disputed, of course), was a heavy user of antacids.

7 Excitotoxins, The Taste that Kills, Blaylock, Russell L., M.D. Health Press, P.O. Drawer 1388 C Santa Fe, NM, 87504, 1945, ISBN 0-929173-14-7.

cury was causing dental patients horrific diseases the ADA denied.

The suppression of the information in this book about mercury has been going on throughout the world in the dental community for more than 160 years even though mercury's poisonous properties have been known for centuries. Everything in this book is well known to the "good old boys—the guys that run the show" in the dental schools and at the ADA. Certainly toxicologists recognize mercury is a very toxic substance. The huge pharmaceutical conglomerates that produce dental amalgam all know. How could they not know? Socrates and Plato reported mercury's poisonality in 400 B.C. The Romans sentenced criminals to work in the cinnabar (mercury) mines of Spain. They had a life expectancy of three years. That is the same poison dentists put in the mouths of our children.

Breach of Trust

For years toxicologists have been trying to inform the public that mercury is a deadly poison.[8] The Toxicology Society has published dozens of research papers about mercury toxicity. Unfortunately, the ADA has enough economic-political power to shut down the very experts they should be listening to. If the ADA would do that, they are certainly not going to inform the public that mercury does not belong in anyone's mouth.

It is inconceivable that in 1992 three thousand physicians and researchers from the Toxicology Society met in Seattle, Washington, to condemn the use of mercury-amalgam dental fillings and there was barely a mention of it in the press. Their revelations should have made banner headlines all around the world. The president of the Toxicology Society told me, "Don't blame the doctors. We teach it to our students. The use of mercury is an economic-political decision."

---

8 The only more poisonous element in the Periodic Table than mercury is plutonium

Dr. Roger Eichman (retired) spent 26 years in private practice. He served on the Alaska Board of Dental Examiners and is a past member of the Board of Directors of the Alaska Miners Association. His expertise is in the field of Industrial Mercury Hygiene and Exposure

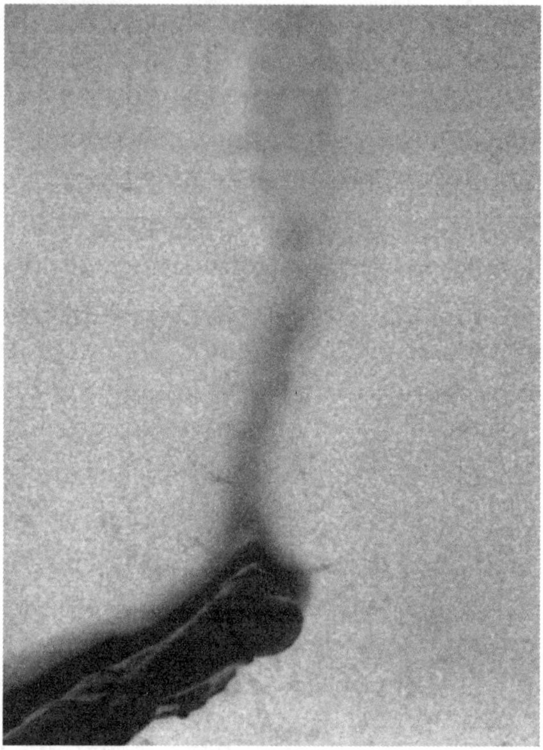

University of Washington
Health Sciences Photography, 2002

The silver filling in Dr. Eichman's forceps is 50 years old. It has been heated to 98.6° (body temperature) and abrased by scratching the top of the filling with a pocketknife. Rubbing an eraser on this filling caused an identical release of mercury vapor. Chewing tobacco, drinking hot coffee or eating hot foods causes more mercury to be released than shown in this photograph, because every 10° C rise in the temperature of mercury doubles the release of mercury.

"Dental vaporization is particularly dangerous due to its closeness to the brain and mercury's ability to cross the blood-brain barrier. The close proximity of the mouth and the brain demands that dentistry pay close attention to brain/dental interactions. Therefore, the use of dental materials must be examined for potential neurotoxicity."

– Dr. Roger Eichman

The dental filling pictured above is a fair comparison to my average mercury amalgam dental filling. The Jerome® Mercury Vapor Analyzer[9] indicated 22 micrograms of mercury were released at body temperature. High-copper dental fillings, in use since 1974, release

9 See Appendix IX for further information about the Jerome Mercury Vapor Analyzer.

mercury up to 50 times faster than seen in this photograph. Washington State environmental protection laws prohibit businesses from exposing workers to more than 100 micrograms of mercury in an eight-hour period. I had 26 dental fillings. Twenty-two times the 26 amalgam fillings I had equal 572 micrograms of mercury vapor exposure in eight hours. Every 24 hours 1,716 micrograms of mercury poisoned me for 35 years.

Economic-Political Decisions

Governments responding to large-scale social, military or economic issues often make decisions that affect the health and welfare of individuals.

Soldiers Exposed to Atomic Bomb Fallout

Every older person in the United States knows that shortly after World War II, American army personnel were placed in shallow trenches not far from a detonation site of an atomic bomb in Nevada. After the blast, they were ordered to maneuver in close proximity to ground zero. Military planners needed to know that if an enemy dropped an atom bomb, would battlefield troops be able to carry out their mission long enough to defeat the enemy? Later, when the former soldiers developed leukemia, lymphoma, melanoma and Hodgkin's disease, some of them tried to bring legal action against the government. Their claims were denied.

Cancer at Hanford Nuclear Reservation

The federal government has at last acknowledged that radioactive materials at Hanford Nuclear Reservation in Washington State caused a number of employees to develop cancer. Sixty years after the fact, most of the older population of workers who suffered lethal radiation exposure are dead. There are many other examples of economic-political decisions that I might have used, but on January 28, 2000, then

Energy Secretary Bill Richardson said, "This is the first time the government is acknowledging workers got cancer from radiation exposure in the plants." On February 3, 2000, the editorial staff of the Seattle Post-Intelligencer newspaper put it this way: "The government has either deliberately deceived its nuclear workers about the health dangers it exposed them to or it has been unconscionably negligent in protecting them." Other similar examples are The Tuskegee syphilis study, Agent Orange and the Gulf War Syndrome cover-up.

The Tuskegee Syphilis study

The Tuskegee syphilis study is another sickening can of worms. It began in the 1920s as an effort by the U.S. Public Health Service to treat low-income black men in Alabama for syphilis, but was converted in 1932 to an experiment to find out what happens when syphilis victims go untreated. The 399 men were kept in the program on the pretense that they were receiving treatment until 1972, when the U.S. Center for Disease Control finally admitted what was going on and the experiment was discontinued. To the unending shame of the scientific community, this reluctant disclosure was no surprise because parts of the research had been published in scientific literature for years.

Agent Orange

Agent Orange, a 50-50 mix of herbicides 2,4-D and 2,4,5-T, was used extensively in Vietnam to defoliate vegetation to prevent enemy troops from ambushing our infantry and to deny the North Vietnamese their hiding places. Agent Orange was sprayed indiscriminately on soldiers and civilians alike and has caused severe health problems for thousands of servicemen and their families. For years the federal government denied Agent Orange was a health hazard even though the manufacturer paid a $180 million out-of-court settlement in a class action lawsuit.

Gulf War Syndrome

Thimerosal[10] (49% mercury) used as a preservative in inoculations, chronic low-level mercurial poisoning from dental fillings plus mercury vapor and cyanide out-gassing from oil wells Saddam Hussein set on fire could be the underlying cause of Gulf War Syndrome. Mercury poisoning causes innumerable symptoms of disease that are subtle and difficult to diagnosis.

Read the Eighth Edition[11] of Goodman and Gilman's *The Pharmacological Basis of Therapeutics* about mercury poisoning and *Recovery From Gulf War Disease* by Dr. Huggins.[12]

Low-level Poisoning from Mercury-Amalgam Dental Fillings

Unfortunately, mercury amalgam has been the dental material of choice for military personnel and their families, welfare recipients, prisoers

---

10 *Facts and Comparisons*, a pharmaceutical reference by Wolters & Kluwer, July, 1992, p 635 and January, 2000, p 1624: Mercury Compounds: Thimerosal (49% mercury) Precautions: For external use only. Avoid contact with the eyes...frequent or prolonged use or applications to large areas may cause serious mercury poisoning.

11 Goodman and Gilman's 9th Edition's information about mercury poisoning appears to have been compromised. In addition, the suggested chelation information is outdated by recent research of Dr. Boyd Haley. If the patient exhibits signs of neurological disease or mental symptoms, i.e., brain-fog or has a nasty disposition, do not use liquid chelation agents. Chemical chelation releases too many heavy metals into the brain that synergistically destroy brain tissue. The trick in recovering from heavy metal poisoning is getting the heavy metals out of the body without killing the patient or flushing his or her I.Q. down the toilet. Drive metal directly to the skin. See "Getting Well Again" in Chapter 3. No disrespect to Goodman and Gilman is intended. They publish the most accurate reference of its type that I've been able to find in the library.

12 See Appendix X.

and hospitalized mental patients longer than I have lived. The federal government unwittingly became embroiled in the ADA's cover-up, because it cannot afford the political and economic reverberations for allowing mercury dental amalgam to be certified by the FDA. The San Francisco Bar Association reports that mercury-amalgam liability is higher than all the money that exists in the United States. In this case denial is the economic-political decision.

For Sale

September 1999, worldwide, the Boeing Airplane Company had 203,800 employees of whom 83,300 worked in Washington State. Their average annual income was $34,300. Worldwide, Microsoft had 31,575 employees. In Washington 16,726 Microsoft employees' average income, including stock options, was $287,700. At the time I collected these figures, in 1999, the King County Public Library Data Base, "Reference USA," listed 3,615 dentists in Washington. The ADA reported that the average annual income of a dentist in the United States in 1998 was $124,000. An endodontist (a dentist who specializes in doing root canals) earned $196,670. I do not have the figures anymore, because I threw that year's Washington State campaign financing files out with a couple of thousand research papers that were taking up too much space in my filing cabinets; but approximately eight years ago, 3,615 dentists contributed more money to political candidates on both sides of the aisle than either Boeing or Microsoft. Those files are public records. Anyone can verify this information.

Harassment

Those whose incomes and reputations are threatened by these revelations will do their utmost to discount this document. Dr. Hal Huggins, the leading mercury-free dentist in the country, has been mercilessly harassed by the dental industry, which is committed to retention of mercury amalgam as the material of choice.

This was not an isolated incident. With one exception, California, ADA dentists who continue to put their economic interests above their patients' health control every dental board in the United States. They are doing everything within their power to put a lid on information that affects their reputations and their pocketbooks.

"If found guilty of being conscientious and giving honest counsel to the patient about the known dangers of mercury, the dentist faces unending harassment . . . resulting in the loss of his or her dental license. The dentist is forced to be an unwilling and silent co-conspirator in the poisoning of his patients.

"In Colorado, Administrative Law Judge Nancy Conic went so far as to write in one of her rulings that Colorado patients who are aware of the toxicity of mercury and request its removal are also liable for fines and imprisonment." —*Dr. Hal Huggins*

To end the harassment, the Colorado legislature passed a law to prevent the ADA from conspiring with their state's dental board and attorney general to put mercury-free dentists out of business. House Bill 97-1187 provides as follows: Section 1, 12-35-118, Colorado Revised Statues, 1991 Repl, Vol., is amended by the addition of a new subsection that says: 1.7 (a) "Nothing in this section shall be construed to deprive any dental patient of the right to choose or replace any professionally recognized restorative material, nor permit disciplinary action against the dentist solely for removing or placing any professionally recognized restorative material."

In 1966, the Chief Medical Officer of the European Commission (in reply to her letter) telephoned a student doing her thesis on dental amalgam. After his expected defense of amalgam, she disagreed with everything he said and stated why there was a worldwide conspiracy about the amalgam issue. (1) Millions of people around the world will rush forward holding amalgam responsible for many ailments and start legal action against their dentists. (2) Practically every dentist would have to be retrained. (3) Insurance companies would be wiped out overnight.[13] She said it just boiled down to money and avoidance of financial catastrophe. There was complete shocked silence at the Chief Medical Officer's end of the line and he then agreed with her. He said there would be a worldwide (economic) catastrophe if the truth about amalgam were known.

Grease

Personal experience within my own industry, insurance, has provided keen insight into corporate contributions to associations or societies. Chief executive officers will hesitate to use corporate profits for research or products that do not pursue the corporate interest. Whenever conglomerates subsidize major expenses of any association, especially those organizations outside of their specific industry, more often than not, the impelling motivation for laying cash on the table is to protect the corporate interest or to make money. For example, the pharmaceutical industry is a major contributor to the Multiple Sclerosis Society. Some pharmaceutical conglomerates produce silver amalgam. Other pharmaceutical corporations spin off their amalgam-manufacturing operations in an effort to separate themselves from legal liability. The Multiple Sclerosis Society continues to deny any connection between silver amalgam dental fillings and MS. I have seen too many people recover from MS after removing their amalgam fillings to believe the MS Society stand. I think they are wrong.[14]

---

13 The author has a certain naivetè about the insurance industry's legal liability.

14 See Appendix VI.

Childhood Vaccinations and Autism

According to Dr. Hugh Fudenberg, one of the world's leading immunogeneticists and 13th most quoted biologist of our times (over 850 peer-reviewed research papers in medical journals), if an individual has had five consecutive flu shots between 1970 and 1980 (the years studied), the chance of getting Alzheimer's disease is ten times higher than if the person had one, two or no flu shots.[15,16]

"Thimerosal, a synonym for mercury, is used as a preservative in injectible vaccines and liquid injectible vitamins, which build up in the brain causing cognitive dysfunction that is expected to cause Alzheimer's to quadruple according to the Johns Hopkins newsletter."[17] Dr. Haley, head of the chemistry department at the University of Kentucky and the internationally recognized researcher on the toxicity of mercury compounds, says, "No amount of thimerosal is a safe amount. Giving a ten-pound infant a single vaccine in a day is the equivalent of giving a 100-pound adult 40 vaccines in a day."

Michael Belkin, president of the National Vaccine Information Center, says, "In the vaccine industry, scientific fraud and conflicts of interest are causing a cycle of deaths and injuries that are being concealed and denied by regulators and vaccine manufacturers."

Parents need to be aware that mercury bioaccumulates in pregnant women's bodies from mercury dental fillings, from fish (especially large bottom fish, shellfish, tuna fish, shark, swordfish, mackerel and tilefish) and that mercury in breast milk and vaccines is often the last of a cumulative number of exposures a baby or toddler is subjected to that synergistically cause autism. A pregnant woman should never go to the dentist, except to have a tooth pulled, until her infant stops

---

15 Recorded from Dr. Fudenberg's speech at the NVIC International Vaccine Conference, Arlington, VA, September 1997. Used with permission.

16 http://autism.about.com/library/weekly/aa092700a.htm

17 Johns Hopkins Newsletter, November 1998.

breast-feeding. It is not well known, but dead brain tissue is found in the spinal fluid for 24 hours after mercury dental filling has been replaced. Even electric toothbrushes cause excessive amounts of mercury to be released from amalgam fillings. The most accurate, up-to-date and informative Web site for medical professionals about the Thimerosal connection to autism is http://www.altcorp.com.

A recent scientific study in the peer-reviewed medical journal, Neurotoxicology, demonstrates mercury, as used in vaccines (Thimerosal), is toxic to proteins, which are indispensable to the human brain. An abstract of that study, "In Vitro Treatment of a Neuroblastoma Cell Line with Low Concentrations of Thimerosal Results in Apoptosis and Altered Nucleotide Binding," will be found in Appendix XII.

The January 2002 *Reader's Digest* has a story entitled "Something's Not Right," which discusses infantile spasms. I carefully compared the symptoms of infantile spasms to the well-documented symptoms of Thimerosal (mercury) poisoning which causes autism and Alzheimer's disease as well as symptoms I still experience that mimic infantile spasms. If I were a betting man, I'd take odds that the most likely cause of infantile spasms is the combination of Thimerosal from childhood vaccines, the mercury secreted in mother's milk and the in-utero exposure to mercury of a fetus from its mother's amalgams. The lack of federal research to examine total mercury exposure by these infants (as well as vaccine-injured infants) is truly a national scandal.

The medical community will undoubtedly meet my speculation about the cause of infantile spasms with derision. However, it was a similar common-sense observation that stopped the needless deaths of thousands of women from childbirth fever in the second half of the 19th century.

Ignaz Semmelweis (1818-1865)

The play "Semmelweis,"[18] which had its world premiere at the National Theatre in Oslo in 1969, has taken on a new relevance due to its chilling parallels with the various scandals surrounding the initial research into AIDS, an epidemic of similar proportions to that of "childbed fever." In the reckless actions of the political and medical authorities in the play, one discerns the same mentality of present-day medical authorities who refused to mandate testing of the blood supply in the United States even though they knew some portion of that supply was contaminated with the AIDS virus. People who think this is a new and unusually complex medical issue, without precedent, and that such political maneuvering can legitimately be excused, need only to reacquaint themselves with the career of this "hero in retrospect," Ignaz Semmelweis.

Dr. Semmelweis was a Hungarian physician who served in the maternity ward of the Vienna Lying-in Hospital where indigent women came for obstetrical care. At the time, one in four mothers died of sepsis infection (childbirth fever). Dr. Semmelweis observed that midwives had a lower sepsis infection rate than medical students (who did autopsies) and suspected that washing hands before delivery might stem the transmission of disease from the cadaver to their patients. He ordered medical students to soak their hands in chlorinated lime before examining pregnant women or delivering babies, and mortality rates for medical students fell to the same level as midwives. For his discovery that the unclean hands of the doctors themselves spread sepsis infection, Dr. Semmelweis was ridiculed by his colleagues, hounded by the police, fired from his position at the Vienna General Hospital, had his works banned, and finally was driven into exile and madness.

---

18 *Semmelweiss* - A play by Jens Bjorneboe, translated from the Norwegian by Joe Martin. Sun and Moon Press, 1999. ISBN: 1557 133508.

Modern-day examples of similar behavior by the dental profession can be found in *Integrity Verses Intimidation* by Dr. Hal Huggins and *Uninformed Consent* by Dr. Hal Huggins and Dr. Thomas Levy. If you have root canals, read *The Root Canal Cover-Up* by Dr. George Meinig. Dr. Meinig was one of the original 19 founding members of the American Association of Endodontists (root canal specialists). A revealing example of the connection between the pharmaceutical-military complex is found in *Emerging Viruses: AIDS & Ebola, Nature, Accident or Intentional* by Dr. Leonard Horowitz.

The Menace of Mercury Thermometers

Better Homes and Gardens, September 2000: "The cities of Ann Arbor, Michigan; Duluth, Minnesota; and San Francisco have recently banned the sale of mercury thermometers for health and environmental reasons. Exposure to mercury in the air and water can cause paralysis, insomnia and delayed development in small children. It also contributes to pollution. One half gram of mercury, the same amount of mercury in most fever thermometers and in one average dental filling, can contaminate all the fish in a 10-acre lake."

The largest pharmacy chains in the United States have discontinued selling mercury thermometers. Our January 2002 utilities bill warned customers not to throw thermometers in the garbage because it adds huge amounts of mercury to the landfill.

Walgreen's, CVS, Rite-Aid, Wal-Mart, Eckerd (J.C. Penney), Albertson's, Kmart, Safeway, Winn-Dixie, Ahold USA, Target, Longs Drug Stores, Costco and Brooks Pharmacy chains have phased out mercury thermometers. In other words, 25,000 pharmacies have discontinued selling mercury thermometers. It is no wonder pharmacists have the reputation for being the most respected group in the medical profession.

During the 2002 legislative session, the Washington State Department of Ecology tried to introduce legislation, as did 24 other states, to stop manufacturers from using mercury in industrial products and force polluters to clean up mercury emissions from industries that contaminate the environment. Not a mention was made about forcing dentists to clean up their act. The Ecology Department knew dentists would scuttle the bill. It seems ludicrous to clean up environmental mercury when two thirds of all the mercury humans are exposed to originate from dental fillings and vaccines.

Where are the Doctors?

There could be another reason the cure for schizophrenia and Alzheimer's disease remains elusive throughout the traditional medical community. The medical profession continues to shirk its responsibility to denounce mercury-silver amalgam dental fillings.

On the surface it appears the American Medical Association has been the ADA's reluctant silent partner for more than 140 years. It also appears that a symbiotic relationship seems to exist between the ADA and AMA. Assuming the word "reluctant" is correct, why would the AMA be so quick to discredit and revoke the medical licenses of physicians who support dentists who inform dental patients that mercury is a carcinogen, a mutagen and a neurotoxin,[19] that mercury doesn't belong in the mouth and amalgams might be the origin of the patient's ill health? Medical doctors have long known Mad Hatter's Syndrome (schizophrenia) was caused by mercury. In the beginning, physicians had a real donnybrook-slugging match with tradesmen-dentists who promoted mercury. The word "quack" is derivative of the German word quicksilver (mercury). Physicians in the 18th century called dentists who used mercury quacks!

So far, I am not prepared to say medical specialists are making a good living off dentists. Later perhaps, if physicians continue to be ambiguous about the amalgam issue, I might have other things to say. For now, let's see how the AMA handles this issue. It's time for doctors to disentangle themselves from the amalgam issue.

---

19 Physicians who may not be aware of the amalgam issue and need definite proof of these accusations should read Section II.

Otherwise

I was in the insurance business 24 years and know what negates liability. When the huge amalgam and root canal class action lawsuits reach the courts, the insurance industry will have little difficulty extricating itself from legal liability because it's a no-brainer to prove the ADA and the American Association of Endodontists (AAE) have committed fraud. Fraud negates liability. Insurance companies will not even be required to return the premiums. Dentists and their supporters will, from a legal position, be as exposed as "The Emperor Who Wore No Clothes." The mercury issue is a hot potato and attorneys like to invite everyone, especially those with deep pockets, to their parties. This is one shindig the AMA ought not attend. The hangover will be a doozy.

Depending on whose toes are getting squished, the answers to the identical health questions from different medical specialists can be poles apart. Each doctor sees the issue through his or her own paradigm, and it is difficult to be objective about information that threatens the pocketbook of a whole trade association, the ADA, which has been in business since 1859.

Disinformation has been spread in both the allergy and dental amalgam issues. In allergy, environmental allergists and traditional allergists joined forces to persuade Washington state politicians to pass legislation that put proponents of the Rasp test, a simple, effective and inexpensive food allergy test, out of business. Plainly, the Rasp test threatened their income. In this same vein the ADA recently published two disingenuous research papers about the safety of mercury-silver amalgam dental fillings. If bona fide scientific research indicates certain substances or products are hazardous and wealthy corporations are caught with their thumb in the soup, they hire unscrupulous professionals to do designer research to fit a predetermined outcome that obscures the issues. It happens all the time in medicine. Examples of deceptive research can be found in the asbestos, breast implant, dental, pharmaceutical and tobacco industries. Be cautious about accepting at face value medical research funded by those who have a vested interest in the results. For example, Parke Davis, the manufacturer of a discontinued diabetic drug, Rezulin®, paid hefty fees to researchers who were directing a National Institutes of Health (NIH) diabetes study on the efficacy of its own product.

The *New England Journal of Medicine (NEJM)* has admitted what is called an extraordinary betrayal of its own ethics saying, "Nearly half the editorials and drug reviews published since 1997 were written by researchers with undisclosed financial support from companies marketing the drugs." The *New England Journal of Medicine* has a conflict-of-interest rule that bars researchers with ties to pharmaceutical companies from submitting reviews or editorials about company products. An American Medical Association spokesman said, "They set up an admirable policy and it's a pity they did not follow up on it."

Anecdotal Evidence Doesn't Count

It does not matter how many people recover. These stories do not mean a thing to the traditional medical community. Anecdotal evidence doesn't count. Of course, I did not diagnose myself.[20] Perhaps the four physicians who told me that I had Alzheimer's disease made a mistake? The woman who read the first edition of *Beating Alzheimer's* and wrote to thank me for her 93-year-old mother's recovery must have been a fluke. Everyone knows Alzheimer's is incurable. The medical profession continually tells the public no one has ever recovered from Alzheimer's disease. My story about a former schizophrenic mental patient who was hospitalized more than 35 years and recovered promptly must be snake oil. I didn't show his psychiatrist what to do. He wouldn't have listened to me. A physician who could not practice anymore recovered from Alzheimer's disease in two hours (two hours flat! Don't worry, fellows, he won't go public. He still needs to work.) The woman who was about to be committed

20 My CAT scans can be viewed in my book *Beating Alzheimer's.*

to Western State (mental) Hospital because it was unsafe to leave her home alone must have also been misdiagnosed. Today she is healthier than I am. Her short-term memory is probably better than her physician's. An Alzheimer's patient lying on her back in a nursing home was taken off the Alzheimer's ward on a stretcher fully recovered. Another woman who was in a coma from low-level mercurial poisoning for 100 days woke up eight days after several amalgam fillings were removed. A young lady was so physically and mentally ill from two titanium posts implanted into her jawbone to hold her lower false teeth in place that her physician told that me she was losing the patient by the hour. After the titanium implants were removed, she recovered.

The Placebo Effect

The anecdotal evidence of tens of thousands of former environmental allergy patients and mercury-free dental patients who have recovered is not considered irrefutable scientific proof connecting mercury, toxic chemicals, food allergy and pollens to brain allergy or chronic disease.

There is the placebo effect to be considered and some validity to suspect emotional illness triggers allergic reactions in hypochondriacs with compromised immune systems. There are reports of cancer going into remission for long periods of time because patients believed the remedy they sought would cure their disease only to die within days after it was announced the treatment proved to be ineffective. A schizophrenic mental patient with multiple personalities exhibited severe allergies in one personality while showing no signs of distress in a different personality. Another schizophrenic and diabetic mental patient exhibited dissimilar blood-glucose levels in separate personalities, which is clear evidence of a mind-body connection to vibrant health or to disease. Scientists and medical professionals should be skeptical of anecdotal evidence in medicine. All the same, after so many anecdotal stories are presented suggesting a reasonable approach to cause and treatment of many ailments, it is time for the medical profession to step back and take a look at the view through a larger picture window.

Could the ADA be lying?

Physicians who are unfamiliar with the ADA mercury-amalgam issue will have a difficult time accepting the information in this paragraph at face value. Temporarily set your preconceptions aside. By the time you finish reading this book, you may feel somewhat differently. Keep in mind that mercury, the main ingredient of a dental filling, is one of the most toxic heavy metals in the Periodic Table. Think the unthinkable: What if one of the leading causes of leukemia and many other forms of cancer, as well as schizophrenia, Alzheimer's, multiple sclerosis, Parkinson's, amyotrophic lateral sclerosis and arteriosclerosis within the heart and the arteries of the brain are symptomatic of a specific iatrogenic disease? If that were true, if you caused those diseases, would you tell on yourself?

One of the foremost chemical references in the world, Sax's Dangerous Properties of Industrial Materials, lists mercury as a possible carcinogen. How is it that dentists tell their patients that mercury—the same substance the Environmental Protection Agency (EPA) calls "hazardous waste" for which strict rules for handling and disposing of—is safe in our mouths less than two inches from our brain? The two concepts, safe and hazardous waste, are incompatible.

Conventional dentists are externally exposed to mercury at least eight hours every working day. Most of them have mercury amalgam fillings in their mouths. Many of them have root canals. Except for the fact that dentists have the highest suicide rate of any professional group,[21] on the surface the majority of dentists do not seem to be particularly troubled by ill health. Since dentists use all kinds of toxic

21 One of the leading side effects of chronic low-level mercurial poisoning is endogenous depression.

heavy metals and chemicals, they seem to develop a cavalier attitude toward these products. Perhaps dentists who still place mercury fillings don't believe the research. Why would they be willing to poison children? Nobody would poison a child for any amount of money. More likely, they just look at the tooth, not the repercussions of the dental materials they use in their practice.

The fact that mercury is strong, durable and easy to use, and initially costs less than gold, does not justify its use. That argument is like curing a headache with cyanide. In fact, gold is cost-effective because of its long, useful life.[22] The amalgam issue is coming down to the wire, fellows. One of the most powerful trial lawyers in the United States, Gerry Spence, says: "Some of the pharmaceutical conglomerates have started to spin off their amalgam operations." It's a legal maneuver to walk away with their bank accounts intact, but that is just not going to happen. Time is running out for amalgam manufacturers and dentists who still place mercury fillings to avoid the legal repercussions.

Perception of Reality

Our perception of reality occurs so naturally and spontaneously that we give little thought to how our brain interprets sight, motion, colors, sound, temperature, odor, touch and pain, etc. It is evident, as we look at any panoramic view, that thousands of synapses and neurons within the brain are working together to differentiate between dissimilar objects, the space between, height, width, depth, and their relationship to one another. Looking out the window, I see different trees, space between green leaves, blue sky, sunlight, clouds, multicolored autumn leaves, and thousands of branches. I hear an automobile passing below my line of sight. It is early in the morning and my hands and feet are cold. Tiffany McGillicutty, our longhaired gray cat, just jumped from the printer to the windowsill. This whole ka-

22 On average, gold filling lasts 11-16 years. The useful life of a mercury amalgam filling is 8.5 years.

leidoscope of information is put together by chemical-electrical energy that flows through brain synapses and neurons constantly interacting with one another. If anything should interfere with the transmission of data along the synapses or between neurons, mixed-up signals might cause stammering, illegible handwriting or distort one's perception of reality causing dyslexia, attention deficit disorder, paranoia, hallucinations, schizophrenia, short-term memory loss or simply cause one to become tired or morose. One might become frightened, tense, grumpy and disruptive, slightly inhibited, or display impulsive, thoughtless, antisocial behavior.

At first glance it seems inconceivable that a single toxic substance could possibly cause so many separate symptoms. But what mercury poisoning does is overwhelm the immune system and poison the brain, the neurological tissue and every cell in the body. In the last 70 years, 208 separate diseases have been linked to mercury-amalgam dental fillings.

What if it could be proved by reproducible scientific research that thought process is inexorably intertwined with heavy metal poisoning, food allergy and environmental chemicals?

Education or ignorance, one's character, a healthy view of life, neurosis, hormones,[23] and emotions influence the choices we select. On the other hand, heavy metal poisoning, food allergy and chemical sensitivity are as connected to inappropriate behavior, schizophrenia and Alzheimer's disease as wind is to a hurricane.

An Introduction to Environmental Medicine

There is an old saying among allergists: "Allergies do not cause everything, but they can cause anything."

23 See *Our Stolen Future*, Theo Colburn, Dumanoski D, Meyers P, Plume, New York 1997.

One of my physicians, Dr. Theron Randolph,[24] was the foremost environmental allergy physician of his time. During his career, Dr. Randolph treated approximately 6,700 cerebral allergy patients who exhibited symptoms that psychiatrists and neurologists would normally diagnose as schizophrenia or the beginning stages of dementia and/or Alzheimer's disease. At least 60 percent, more than 4,000, were cured without pharmaceutical medications or further medical intervention. Dr. Randolph was unpopular in traditional medical circles because he was able to cure more than 15,000 patients from dozens of chronic diseases that mainstream medical doctors believed to be incurable. Dr. Randolph told me his patients had seen, on average, 25 traditional medical doctors before seeking his services.

Most of us, myself included, were near the end of our tether. All of us were chronically ill or dying. Without taking anything away from this great man, at the time I was Dr. Randolph's patient, he was unfamiliar with the amalgam issue or the connection between low-level mercurial poisoning, low HCl (stomach acid) and of the digestive enzyme connection to cerebral allergy, as well as the mentally ill patient's need for vitamin and mineral supplementation. Dr. Randolph had met Dr. William Crook, the author of *The Yeast Connection*, and started his food allergy patients on nystatin to clear up candida albican yeast overgrowth. The important thing Dr. Randolph did do was to teach his chronically ill patients how to identify favorite foods, chemicals in or on foods, and other environmental chemicals and pollens that cause many allergy sufferers chronic disease and/or brain-fog.[25]

If I had not become Dr. Randolph's patient, attended his classes and learned everything that he was willing to teach us during my stay in his Environmental Allergy Unit, this book could not have been written because I would have died many years ago from Alzheimer's disease.

Dr. Richard Wilkerson of Yakima, Washington; David Buscher of

---

24 Dr. Theron Randolph (1906-1995) of Chicago.

Bellevue, Washington; Dr. Bill Ray of Dallas, Texas; and so many other protégés of Dr. Randolph have taken his understanding of environmental medicine so much further. Dr. Sandra Denton,[26] of Anchorage, Alaska, treats allergy patients (most of whom have been poisoned by low-level mercurial toxicity from mercury amalgam dental fillings) in an entirely different way than Dr. Wilkerson, Dr. Buscher or Dr. Ray. Her treatment protocol is every bit as effective, in fact, more so. (I will disclose her treatment procedures later.) Dr. Hugh Fudenberg, a neuroimmunologist from Spartanburg, South Carolina, uses the "Transfer Factor"[27] among other modalities of traditional treatment. His methodology requires such exactitude in producing the transfer factor that the average physician would not be able to do it. Dr. Fudenberg is in a class all by himself. These physicians are among the giants of today that Dr. Randolph was during his career.

Do not become impatient, keep reading: All this information leads directly to the cause and cure for many chronic diseases.

Stressors

Chronic low-level mercury poisoning weakens the immune system and leaves the door open to a whole host of opportunistic diseases.

Let's suppose your grandparents were farmers who lived long and happy lives. Their immune systems might be compared to a huge European wine vat. During World War II, food processors introduced chemicalized foodstuffs to store for long periods of time in many dif-

---

25 Spaced-out feeling: a person becomes somewhat dissociated from reality, as if they stood ten or twelve feet off in the fog viewing what's going on as a spaced-out, troubled or disinterested third person. For all intents and purposes they are not in touch with reality. At that point they need to crash in their "clean room" until their thinking clears. The clean room (the oasis) is covered in chapter three.

26 Sandra Denton's office telephone number is (907) 563-6200.

27 It is possible to transfer immunity to cerebral allergies from a healthy person to Alzheimer's patients.

ferent climates. Our military were spread throughout Europe, Asia, the Atlantic Ocean and Pacific theaters, and foods were packaged to accommodate that situation, but the chemicalization of foods had a cost: it placed new limits on the human immune system. So your father and mother's immune systems might be compared to a rain barrel. If your family had chronic disease like mine, your immune system might be compared to a bucket.

Stressors can be almost anything: eating your favorite foods too often, cosmetics—especially hair spray—chlorine, automotive exhaust, heavy metal poisoning, toxic environmental chemicals, pollens, molds, junk food, neurosis, burning the candle at both ends, a job that's wearing you down, a marriage that's falling apart, financial problems, candle wicks that out-gas lead, inadequate housing, a death in the family. Now, take any number of stressors and throw them one-by-one into the wine vat, the rain barrel or the bucket. You will not succumb to disease until your container fills and one drop of water spills over the side. That drop of water spilling over the side is like jumping out of an airplane without a parachute. The disease you land on depends on your genetic history. If your ancestors had Alzheimer's disease, that's the square you are most likely to land on. Toxic metals and infectious bacteria seek targets of opportunity, the frailest organs and the weakest genes in our family tree to do their mischief.

The Consequences of Mercurial Poisoning

"The brain succumbs to methyl mercury's ravages more readily than other tissues.

First, mercury damages the brain without appreciable loss of cells (see photo next page) then erodes whole pockets of tissue.

Worst hit the brain's visual, hearing and equilibrium centers, thus explaining the effects of mercury poisoning - blindness, deafness and loss of balance."

—James Stanfield and Robert Madden, the *National Geographic*, "Quicksilver and Slow Death," October 1972.

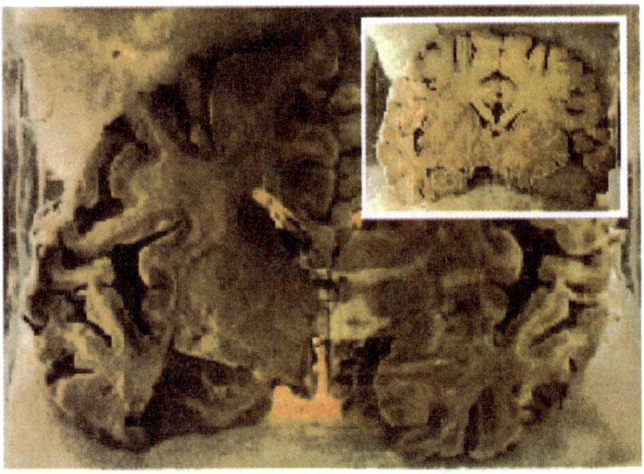

(Inset picture above shows normal brain tissue. Larger picture shows brain with mercury damage.)

In the absence of obvious physical illness or injury, heavy metal poisoning, root canals, jawbone infection, toxic chemical exposure, food allergy, and poor nutrition should be considered as possible underlying causes of endogenous depression, aberrant and/or abrasive behavior, schizophrenia, Alzheimer's disease and dysfunctional family development. If the above statement can be proved, it is the key to curing millions of mentally ill nonconformists on our streets, hospitalized mental patients, and sociopaths in our jails and prison system. Why would anyone think that toxic metals and environmental chemicals that synergistically poison the brain would not cause erratic behavior?

The Food Allergy Toxic Chemical Connection to Irrational Behavior

Roughly 30 percent of Alzheimer's sufferers become irritable due to heavy metal poisoning and exposure to chemicals in products such as hair spray, underarm deodorant, perfume, petrochemical newsprint, chlorinated soaps and cleansers, formaldehyde fumes, insect spray,[28] lighted candles,[29] mold, wood or coal-burning stoves, gas or oil fur-

28 Insect spray contains many poisons, including mercury.
29 The wicks of candles out-gas lead. A burning candle reduces oxygen.

naces and automotive fumes—especially diesel exhaust[30]— as well as favorite food and pollen allergies.

Forty years ago Father Allen Amirault—Catholic priest, professor, psychologist, hospital chaplain and friend—looked slightly perplexed as he remarked, "There is something we do not understand about mental illness. We think people are a lot more responsible for their actions than they actually are."

There was a program on public television about a truck driver who hauled petroleum. He accidentally caught a strong whiff of gasoline additive as he topped off the tanker and for the next couple of days had an urgent need to urinate. He was driving along a busy street when it became impossible to hold his bladder any longer. In panic, he hurriedly parked his vehicle along the curve and ran across a lawn into the bushes of a nearby house to relieve himself. An agitated woman rushed outside on the veranda to view the spectacle and began calling the fellow vulgar names, whereupon the driver, a man who until that instant had never been in trouble with the law in his life, ran up onto the porch and killed her. Prison psychiatrists recognized a connection between the driver's explosive rage and indirectly suggested chemical sensitivity was the underlying cause of the provoked attack. As you read this book, keep that thought in mind.

There is a story in *5-Day Allergy Relief* about a prison inmate who constantly assaulted other prisoners. Every time he ate eggs, one of his favorite foods, his fists started flying. Almost everyone knows that liquor, street drugs, psychotropic medications, chocolate and excessive amounts of coffee affect human behavior. I predict that some day, prisoners on parole will be held as accountable for their diet and

30 All petrochemical fumes emit trace amounts of mercury and cyanide. I suspect auto exhaust emissions might be connected to road-rage and that out-gassing hydrocarbon fumes from gas stoves are connected to the proverbial nasty disposition of professional cooks. There is a story connecting gas stoves to schizphrenia, and candles to all sorts of medical problems, in *Beating Alzheimer's.*

toxic chemicals to which they knowingly expose themselves as people who commit crimes while intoxicated, or who use street drugs today.

Behind much deviant or violent behavior, the physician can often expect to find heavy metal and/or chemical poisoning, food allergy and nutritional deficiencies. If the patient has several mercury dental fillings, then expect also to find low-normal thyroid, low enzyme production and low stomach acid. Expect the psychiatric community to say, "We can't deal with all that." What I suggest—removal of amalgams and avoidance of mercury and other environmental toxins—is far less expensive, time-consuming and troublesome than taking psychotropic pharmaceuticals, or years upon years of psychotherapy that goes nowhere. If psychotherapy takes longer than three years to cut to the core of the patient's distress, cerebral allergies are most likely confusing the issue. It is possible to stop uncharacteristic behavior faster than family members, psychologists and psychiatrists or law-enforcement officials realize.

A woman at her wit's end narrated a litany of her son's conduct to William Walsh, PhD, director of the Carl Pfeiffer Treatment Center.[31] The more the mother went on with the account of her son's reprehensible activities, the more Dr. Walsh's face brightened into a smile. She hit the roof and demanded to know why Dr. Walsh appeared to be in high spirits while her world was falling apart. Dr. Walsh replied, "Because your son's appalling behavior indicates that he is someone we can help. He will recover."

The government sent hair and tissue samples from mass-murderers to be analyzed by Dr. Walsh's laboratory. With one exception, they all had high levels of heavy metal toxicity. However, one convict had the lowest level of copper Dr. Walsh had ever seen. The connection between mercury amalgam toxicity and aberrant abrasive behavior has been shown in clinical studies. The following abstract is a prime ex-

---

31 Carl Pfeiffer Treatment Center and Health Resource Institute, 1894 Centre Pointe Drive Suite 106, Naperville, IL 60563 (630) 505-0300.

ample: "Potential toxicity from exposure to mercury from dental amalgam fillings is the subject of current public health debate in many countries."[32]

Mercury

Read the mercury Material Safety Data Sheets (MSDS) sheets in Section II. Due to copyright infringement laws, I am prevented from quoting the MSDS sheets in their entirety. However, they discuss many medical problems caused by mercury other than mental disease.

For a graphic demonstration of the harm caused to the brain by mercury: If you have a newer computer with at least 128 megabytes of ram, go to http://movies.commons.ucalgary.ca/mercury. The streaming video is five minutes long. No one who reads the first three MSDS sheets at the start of Section II, and views the University of Calgary's Neuroscience video entitled *How Mercury Causes Neurodegeneration* of the brain, will allow a dentist to put a mercury dental filling in his or her mouth again.

Lead

The major symptoms of lead poisoning are endogenous depression, headaches, and mood swings, poor concentration, learning difficulties, confusion, memory problems, irritability, agitation and violence. Compare those symptoms with the signs of mercury toxicity in Appendix I. Anyone who has ever lived in an older home has some degree of lead poisoning from solder in old plumbing and lead in old paint.

On January 19, 2002, there was a story in the *New York Times* by Jodi Wilgoren entitled "Poison Covers Missouri Town Like a Lead Blanket." The article tells how lead exposure from the Doe Run Company Smelter and huge piles of slag poisoned Herculaneum, Missouri. Phy-

32 See Appendix XII.

sicians found high levels of lead in the blood of 25 percent of the town's children under 6. What a bleak future these children face. March 23, 2002, the *Seattle Post-Intelligencer* carried a story from Associated Press by David Scott entitled "Lead Risk Prompts Buyout. Smelter to start with homes of children under 6."

The Synergistic Effect of Mercury and Lead

One lethal dose (LD 1) means 1 dose of any poison that kills one rat in 100. The synergistic effect of combining 1 LD mercury (Hg) and 1 LD lead (Pb) equals LD 100. All 100 rats die.[33] LD 50 is considered toxic to humans. The implications of this information for children living in old housing sloshed with lead paint and lead-soldered water pipes, in conjunction with mercury amalgam fillings, are truly frightening.

Aluminum

Aluminum (Al) poisoning from pots and pans, antacids, underarm deodorants, and aluminum sulfate used to treat drinking water causes mood swings and mental retardation. A University of Kentucky study reported that some Alzheimer's cadavers had high levels of aluminum in their brains. Recent research by the University of Calgary neuroscience team rules out aluminum by itself, as causing Alzheimer's disease.

"The aluminum industry is gathering together all research documents, marketing promotion documents and trade association documents for that near future time when individual populations worldwide will wake up to the dangers of its aluminum products. Court actions are inevitable. In the meantime, aluminum company executives are attempting to win friends for themselves and the industry. For instance, Edward Truschke,

33 Dr. J. Schubert, *Journal of Toxicology and Environmental Health*, Volume 4-763, 1978. "Combined Effect of toxicity, a rapid testing procedure for cadmium, mercury and lead."

the executive director of the Alzheimer's Association headquartered in Chicago, in response to our multiple inquiries, finally admitted that his organization has received unrestricted grant monies from the Aluminum Association of Canada (ALCAN) and from the Aluminum Company of America (ALCOA). He did not acknowledge, but we are aware that the International Alzheimer's disease medical meeting held July 1992, in Italy, was sponsored in part by the Aluminum Association of Canada."

—Dr. Richard Casdorph and Dr. Morton Walker.[34]

It appears there is a conflict of interest and unethical behavior might be involved, but appearances are often deceiving. This issue needs to be addressed. The Alzheimer's Association's reputation is at stake and I suspect charitable donations will suffer unless this matter is quickly resolved. An audit of the Alzheimer's Association, ALCOA and ALCAN funding would settle the issue.

Copper

Copper (Cu) is an essential mineral in human nutrient in the correct proportions. Insufficient copper causes aneurysms, and has also been traced to deviant behavior. High copper levels in the brain cause endogenous depression, mood swings, irritability, aggressive behavior, low I.Q. scores and dementia.

Water is called the universal solvent. The average concentration of copper in tap water ranges from 20 to 75 copper parts per billion (ppb). However, some new homes have copper concentrations of more than 1000 ppb. That is more than 1 milligram Cu per liter of water. Copper is picked up from copper pipes and brass faucets, especially when the water sits in the pipes overnight. After the water is allowed to run for a while, the concentration of copper in the water decreases. The average running stream in the U.S. has 300 ppb copper. The water on the Sammamish Plateau in Washington State had 1000 ppb at the wellhead; the water from the kitchen faucet of the apartment we

---

34 Dr. Morton Walker verified that this information is accurate.

lived in for a while registered 2000 ppb. In June 1997, a diagnostic urine test revealed that I excreted excessive lead, copper and mercury.

Irrational Behavior

A woman who had been a dental assistant in her youth (think "mercury exposure") became paranoid and suffered from schizophrenia most of her life. While she was lucid, she was a kind, easygoing, articulate person. The woman believed neighbors wished to cause her great harm. After cooking, she often had hallucinations in which she saw invisible people putting "dope" into the food on her plate. She told me "I can prove the food is being doped," because her brother and sister always fought after dinner. That observation indicated that she had more insight into her illness than anyone suspected because, no matter how serene their frame of mind was before dinner, her relatives continually engaged in shouting matches after dinner (food allergy). There was an old coal stove in the kitchen on which the woman used to cook the family meals, and an oil stove in the dining room that discharged obnoxious petrochemical fumes (chemical sensitivity). Coal and petrochemicals discharge mercury vapor and carbon monoxide—lethal poisons. That is the reason local building codes in our area require contractors to install carbon monoxide detectors.

Indoor Air Pollution

"Most physicians tend to overlook indoor air pollution as a cause of dementia in the elderly. Consider the case of a 79-year-old widow who suffered progressive cognitive deterioration after her husband's death. She was diagnosed with Alzheimer's disease and her family made arrangements to place her in a nursing home.

"But by chance, a family friend was a physician and well informed about environmental health effects. In reviewing her case, he cast doubt on the Alzheimer's diagnosis. Despite the grief over losing her husband, she had remained mentally sharp for four months after his death. At that point she sold their home and moved into a new condominium. Her symptoms appeared after living there two months and progressed more quickly than Alzheimer's usually does. Further investigation revealed that she had high blood levels of toluene,[35] a toxic chemical used in construction materials, which contaminates the indoor air of new buildings, even those that appear to be adequately ventilated. On the advice of the environmental physician, the woman moved out of her condo to her daughter's older home. Three weeks later, she was back to her old self."

—Story from http://www.alzheimers.com.au[36]

Pharmaceutical Medications

There is a story in *Beating Alzheimer's* about a woman diagnosed as having Alzheimer's disease who was placed in a nursing home for three years before physicians realized her short-term memory problems were caused by the medications she was taking. The following information is important: Purchase your prescriptions from a single pharmacy, especially if you are seeing more than one physician. If for no other reason than understanding drug interactions, I recommend reading *Beating Alzheimer's*. Ask your pharmacist for a package insert for all of the patient's prescriptions and carefully read the known side effects. Then ask him or her to please check the computer to see if there are drug interactions between the different medications the patient is taking.

Proof that Environmental Toxins Disrupt Thought Process

There is recent solid scientific evidence that toxins disrupt the kaleidoscope of thought processes and distort one's perception of reality —at least in a grasshopper. Before psychiatrists, the chemical industry and the ADA all seek to discount this epic breakthrough in brain research, it should be known that the brains of all animals process

35 Toluene is a component of many products, including cosmetics, paint sprays, paint removers and thinners, correction fluid glue and other products.

36 See Appendix XII for Toluene Research.

information in a manner similar to human beings. If toxins affect the transmission of data traveling along neurons or distort signals between synapses in a grasshopper, toxins affect people in the same way.

Dr. Chris Diorio, a computer scientist at the University of Washington, gave a lecture on University of Washington television to computer students in which he casually mentioned computer-related medical research by Kate MacLeod for her thesis at the Caltech Graduate Study Program in Biology. MacLeod proved that toxins disrupt the signals passing along the synapses within the brain of a live grasshopper. Before a toxin was introduced to the grasshopper, the computer generated reproducible bar codes of energy passing along the grasshopper's synapses similar to the bar code that check stands use to scan prices off a box of cereal in a grocery store. After a toxin was introduced to the grasshopper, the bar code had not changed in intensity; it was exactly the same height as before, but the lines of code had changed. That reaction is similar to the phenomenon that cerebral allergy sufferers experience, that we call brain-fog or brain-fag.[37]

The reason I understand this whole issue so well is that I still deal with cerebral allergies every single day. The reason I am well is due to removing mercury dental fillings and knowing how to decontaminate my living environment and, for the most part, I have learned. which foods and chemicals produce brain-fog or brain-fag. I have seen similar allergic reactions to foods and chemicals in most people who suffer from a variety of chronic diseases.

If I had kept my mercury dental fillings, if I had not had 20 jawbone infections (cavitations) cleaned up within my jawbones, if I had allowed myself to be exposed to formaldehyde fumes and bleaches that use mercury in the manufacturing process... If we had continued to park our automobile under or in a garage connected to our home... If I had not quit using substances containing MSG, EDTA, or other

37 Feeling like a cranky child who needs to take a nap.

excitotoxins[38] that kill brain cells... and if I had not stayed away from dozens of other chemicals and pesticides used in/or on hundreds of foodstuffs, my thought process would have evaporated. I would be as explosive and unpredictable as a plugged-up badger. Before I learned the way through the maze in which I was trapped, no one would have mourned my passing. That type of behavior is predictable pathology for many people suffering from heavy metal and chemical poisoning.

If the reader is concerned with, someone suffering from short-term memory loss, brain-fog, or schizophrenia, the above paragraph is another reason for buying *Beating Alzheimer's*. It not only covers the side effects of pharmaceutical medications better than I will able to write in this book because of copyright infringement; it focuses on the basics of chemical contamination within the home. It is also less comprehensive and easier to understand. At the time I wrote *Beating Alzheimer's*, I was unaware of the multitude of diseases caused by heavy metal poisoning and suspect that no matter how clear I try to write this manuscript, it might be too difficult for Alzheimer's sufferers to deal with. I intend to make the chapter "Getting Well Again" as clear and uncomplicated as is within my power. Alzheimer's sufferers: Keep it simple; stick with Chapter 3, "Getting Well Again." Do not cause yourself more stress than necessary. Read the rest of the book as your thought process clears.

Cerebral allergies and/or chemical sensitivities producing brain-fog are the reason Alzheimer's patients' memories appear relatively normal at times and they are unable to recognize family members the very next day. In particular, exposure to environmental chemicals tends to cause thoughtless, irrational and obnoxious behavior. The good news in all this, assuming your mercury fillings, root canals and cavitations have been correctly removed, is that the road map through the maze of learning how to control brain allergies and undoing the mis-

38 Used as a preservative and flavor enhancer in many dry cereals and baby foods.

chief caused by environmental toxins is doable. It takes a while, and seems overwhelming at first, but it is not particularly difficult to learn the road map through the maze in which the patient seems trapped. The trick is to DO IT, because it takes real tenacity to keep putting one foot ahead of the other when you feel like falling off the ends of the earth.

The Amalgam Debate-A Lawyer's View

By Christopher A. Bomba

"The amalgam debate is both scientific and political. There are highly trained and intelligent experts on both sides. It is not merely a debate between those who understand the scientific method and those who do not. In fact, those who might try to convince you otherwise are using a form of argumentative propaganda. This ploy involves choosing a phrase, scientific method, which has a generally accepted positive connotation, and fortuitously associating oneself with it. The truth is that the scientific method gets used and abused for all manner of ends... An awful lot of people with MD, DDS, and PhD at the ends of their names have concluded that mercury amalgams are dangerous to the dental patient's health. Many others still think they are safe. Thus, we have a growing scientific debate.

It is also important to remember that this debate is political. By political, I mean that there is a lot more at stake than an esoteric scientific idea. Obviously thousands of dentists have their fortunes as well as their self-respect at risk. An entire industry may be disrupted or dismembered if the amalgams are proven dangerous. The manufacturers are only a small part of this industry. This industry is composed of every dentist who has ever potentially poisoned people by implanting mercury in their mouths as well as their lobbyists and their supporters in the medical profession. The ADA would be devastated by the undermining of its credibility, and the Federal Drug Administration would have a heck of a time explaining to the public why it "grandfathered" the use of mercury amalgams without the vigorous proof of safety now required of new devices. There are potentially millions of people who have been harmed. And thus we can see why this debate is so heated.

In the coming decade, as evidence of the danger of mercury amalgams accumulates, we will see an explosion of litigation similar to that associated with asbestos, silicone implants and tobacco cigarettes. Eventually, perhaps in ten to twenty years, mercury amalgams will be banned in the United States. In the meantime, being a prudent and wily lawyer with few other options, I have taken the mounting evidence so seriously as to have my amalgams removed. I am currently engaged in an intensive detoxification program, with some positive results.

We shall see what we shall see."

Christopher Bomba is an attorney experienced in toxic product litigation. His e-mail address is: cabomba@citcom.net

Chapter 2

Jawbone Infection and Systemic Disease

In the late 1880s the root canal issue and the jawbone infection connection to systemic disease was unknown to mainstream dentistry. If one reads the literature, it appears there has been ongoing suppression of the root canal issue and of jawbone infection to chronic disease by the ADA and American Endodontist Association (AEA) since the early 1940s. Dental students will not find *Dental Infections, Oral and Systemic Disease* by Dr. Weston Price in any dental school libraries. It has been taken off the shelves.

In the early 1900s Dr. Frank Billings,[39] who introduced the focal infection theory,[40] asserted that 95 percent of all focal infections in the body comes from decayed teeth and infected tonsils. In the 1920s the National Dental Association[41] appointed Dr. Weston Price and a team of 60 scientists and physicians to do a study that proved bacteria and toxins within dentin tubules[42] of root-canalled teeth and cavita-

39 Dr. Frank Billings: Former Dean of the faculty and Professor of Medicine at the University of Chicago in the early 1900s.

40 Focal Infection. Patho: dentistry. An infection in which bacteria are localized in some region, as around the tooth, to which they may spread to some other organ or structure in the body.

41 The National Dental Association merged with the ADA. Dentin Tubules: The tooth structure is porous and dentin tublules (hollow tubes) within a single tooth are approximately three miles in length.

42 Eight bacteria fit side by side within one dentin tubule, which makes bacteria difficult to eradicate. It is not uncommon for cavitations to become reinfected.

tions[43] (areas of bone necrosis)[44] caused disease.

Dr. Meinig, author of the *Root Canal Cover-Up*, graciously told me the following is how he explains what physicians and others need to know about focal infections.[45]

"The bacteria (microbes and other organisms) present in the dentin tubules due to infection in the cavities that penetrate the pulp find the tubule such a great place to live because in normal health they contain a fluid that has nutrients. Those nutrients are what keep teeth alive and healthy. The nutrients are supplied 24 hours a day, just the same as arteries supply all tissues and cells with nutrients 24 hours a day.

"The fluid in the tubules has movement from the root canal to all parts of the tooth. When the tooth becomes infected, the bacteria are said to be trapped in the tubules but they really aren't. They escape by lateral, accessory root canals to the periodontal membrane, the tough fibrous tissue that holds the tooth in its bony socket.

"The periodontal membrane also has a good blood supply and in turn, as it becomes infected, bacteria are easily transferred to the surrounding bony socket and its blood supply.

"The bacteria can then metastasize,[46] like cancer cells, to any gland, organ or tissue of the body where they set up a whole new focal infection.

"The Endodontists Association says, so what! The immune system will get rid of them, and they are correct, but here's what happens. There are more than

---

43 Cavitations: Infected areas within the jawbone.
44 Bone necrosis: Disease caused to healthy cells due to direct contact with any agent (usually living organism) capable of producing infection.
45 Disease generated from the jawbone infection also metastasizes through the acupuncture median system.
46 Metastasize: the spread of disease from one part of the body to another.

100 active immune system cells that go to work whenever bacteria or toxins appear. Each has the ability to get rid of certain specialized foreign materials.

"Dr. Weston Price, in a study of 5,000 patients, found that those who had excellent genetic backgrounds, what he called good defense systems, could tolerate these bacteria for many years. Price not only studied the health of the patient but also the parent and grandparent. He found that if the grandparents and parents lived long and healthy lives and their siblings were free from disease, they had strong immune systems that they passed along to their children.

"If the dental patient was healthy, Dr. Price did not discourage them from having a root canal. What he found was that most of these patients came under severe stress sometime in their life—an accident, a case of flu, or death of a close family member. Now their immune system that previously protected them so well could no longer do so and they often came down with degenerative disease.

"What Price didn't know, what we have found in these succeeding years, is even when a stress situation had not occurred, sometimes patients still developed degenerative disease.

"It took quite a few years, but the dentists trying to solve these problems found that the bacteria escaping from the dentin tubules 24 hours a day, day after day, week after week, year after year, caused those very efficient immune cells to become tired, worn out, no longer able to perform as before, and the patients' immune systems became so compromised that they finally came down with degenerative diseases.

"Keep in mind that the original disease was focal infection but as the patient's immune system gets knocked out, one of the degenerative diseases takes over. Dr. Price found 20 bacteria were involved in these focal infections. Most were streptococcus, but they could also be staphylococcus, spirochetes or fungi. What happens frequently is that the patient with a worn-out immune system can quite easily become the victim of two or more different degenerative diseases.

"The prime goal of physicians is to try and find the cause of whatever the patient is suffering.

Tom, you are quite aware many different causes prevail. These can be different organisms, nutritional deficiencies, toxins of various kinds from numbers of sources that stress the immune system, e.g., severe working conditions, problems at home or environmental stress, etc.

"But the most prevalent reason of which very few medical practitioners are aware is that teeth or other oral diseases cause 95 percent of all focal infections. Keep in mind that the average dentist and physician is unaware of how much and how often teeth and oral disease are the origin of the patient's illness. Most doctors are oblivious to the fact that teeth are the cause of their patients' degenerative diseases 95 percent of the time. This never becomes a consideration because the medical community just doesn't know the research. Consequently, patients go down hill, do not recover, and end up dying before their time.

"Now you can really see just how important our work is in advising everyone how dangerous root-canal filled teeth, jawbone cavitations, periodontal and other oral diseases are. Oral health is more connected to disease and longevity than anyone suspects." *—Thank you, Dr. Meinig.*

Remember the physician who had retired due to short-term memory loss who had 13 root canals, mentioned in Chapter 1? He read the first edition of *Beating Alzheimer's* and pestered me ad infinitum for further proof that, if he was to have any chance for recovery, he needed to have all of his teeth extracted. The reason for his indecision was the infeasibility of bridging the spaces between 13 root canals. For six months he checked and rechecked with mercury-free dentists and physicians from all over the world, mentioned in my book, before he went ahead. After his teeth were pulled, he went home and lay down expecting to die, but awoke two hours later. He said, "It was the first time in years my head was clear." He has been back in full-time practice for almost a decade.

According to Dr. Gerald Becker[47]:

---

47 Dr. Gerald L. Becker, Highland Park Place, 715 N. 182nd St., Ste 401, Shoreline, WA (206) 542-4848

"These areas of chronic inflammation, infection, cellular disruption and electrical alteration exist in bony cavities in the upper and lower jawbone. They originate from remaining infected tissue left over after tooth extraction.

"After tooth extraction, the socket frequently covers over with a thin layer of bone that appears normal to most dentists. However, inside is a cavernous area lined with dead bone cells, dead fat cells, fibrin sludge, delaminated bone, polymorphonuclear leucocytes (PMNs), dead blood cells and bacteria colonies.

"Most root-filled teeth, when extracted, have a small sac of infected tissue attached. The bone around the cavity must be thoroughly cleaned out to allow healing with normal bone tissue. There can be dramatic effects when root canals and cavitations are removed.[48]

"The relationships between mercury fillings, acupuncture meridians, oral electrical galvanism, root canals, cavitations, heavy metal toxicity and chemical sensitivities are complex and not totally understood by the traditional dental community."

Acupuncture Meridians

Meridians are pathways in the body along which vital energy flows.[49]

John Moore, a friend involved in the amalgam issue, told me about a woman who had a breast tumor. Oncologists (cancer specialists) do not like to operate if there are signs of other infection. Her physician asked the woman to have an abscessed tooth taken care of before surgery. Immediately after the dental appointment, while Lidocaine was still present in her system, the woman had a thermography examination that revealed a thin white line extending from an abscessed tooth, down her neck, through the tumor in her breast and on down into her stomach. In light of the discovery, her physicians decided not

48 Medical professionals, see Appendix XIII for further information.

49 Random House Unabridged Dictionary, Second Edition.

to operate. Four months later, the tumor disappeared. I repeated her story to the late Glen Warner's cancer group a while back. Eighteen months, maybe two years ago, a man pulled on my sleeve and said, "It was providential that they (his wife and himself) came that night because his wife had a breast tumor. She replaced her mercury fillings. Four months later the tumor disappeared and has not returned." John reminded me about one of the fellows who came to several of our seminars. George's arm hung from his shoulder like a hindquarter of beef in a storage freezer. Surgeons operated two times to restore movement in his arm. They planned to do a third operation, but luckily, George learned tooth number 19 had a root canal whose acupuncture meridian ran through his arm muscle. He had an alternative practice dentist pull tooth 19. Within 48 hours full range of motion returned to his arm. It took another six months before his withered arm regained its former strength.

Sometimes cavitations become reinfected. I assumed my thought process was all right, but the instant the dentist's drill breached a hollow reinfected cavitation in my jawbone, my thought processes instantly became crystal clear. I was so taken aback by the exactitude of my clarity that it brought tears to my eyes, and I stepped out of the dental office by the back door to compose myself. This is difficult to write, because I think of myself as being a suck-up-the-gut tough guy and it is embarrassing to admit that under the right circumstances I show emotion. The reason for revealing this information is that the public needs to recognize jawbone infection, all by itself, can cause muddled thinking.

So, if you are considering a root canal instead of an extraction, better give the idea more thought. If you have neurological problems or any other chronic disease and already have root canals—if it were I, I'd have them extracted immediately.

What is apparent is that dental students need more in-depth training about the oral cavity's connection to chronic disease than our dental schools have been providing.

"Although the migration of bacteria and other microorganisms through the acupuncture meridians is not yet scientifically accepted, it seems likely that it will eventually be shown as an important way for focal infections to spread."

— Dr. Richard Gerber

Jawbone infection can damage a person's health at any time. Physicians will find that most chronically ill patients (never mind the disease) have jawbone infection. Until recently there wasn't any way to accurately visualize jawbone infection because cavitations are hollow and x-rays cannot take pictures of air. Cavitat technology has changed all that.

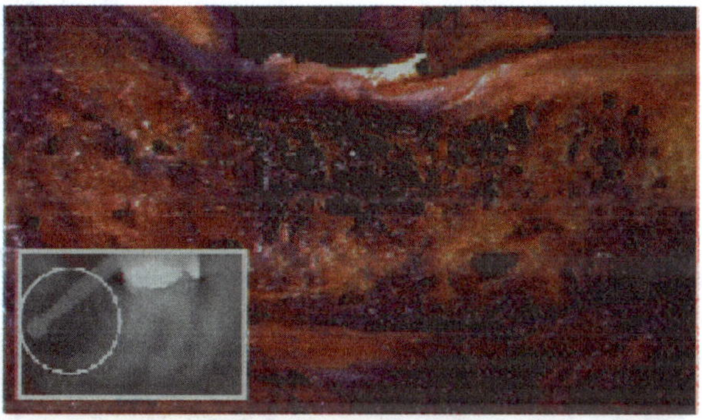

The dental patient does not feel pain until the infection reaches the trigeminal nerve. At that point the pain becomes agonizing and intervention ineffective.

Cavitations are extremely difficult to visualize on x-rays. No cavitations were observed on the x-rays of the above jawbone. The dark areas are infected. In the insert a dentist has placed a dental drill in a cleaned out cavitation to illustrate how deep some cavitations are.

If the dental patient is low on trace minerals or the macro minerals, sodium, potassium, calcium and magnesium pantomography-x-rays are at best, unreliable. I took an original panex-x-ray to the Oral Radiology Department at the University of Washington dental school to be examined. The doctor scrutinized it very, very carefully for approximately ten minutes and couldn't find the slightest sign of infection within my jawbone. The following computer-generated images reveal nine (ischemic osteoporosis) infected cavitations. Four of them, are on the brink of causing serious medical problems.

Tooth and jawbone infection is more connected to chronic disease than the public realizes. In the late 1800's the leading cause of death in Washington State was oral infection. For the dental community to ignore this issue reeks of ignorance and evasion of responsibility.

The Cavitat

"It would be difficult to exaggerate the detail and accuracy with which the Cavitat reveals osteonecrosis in the jaw. It provides not only dental, but also systemic health benefits not previously available."

—Dr. Boyd Haley

The Cavitat[50] is an acoustic sound-wave diagnostic instrument that

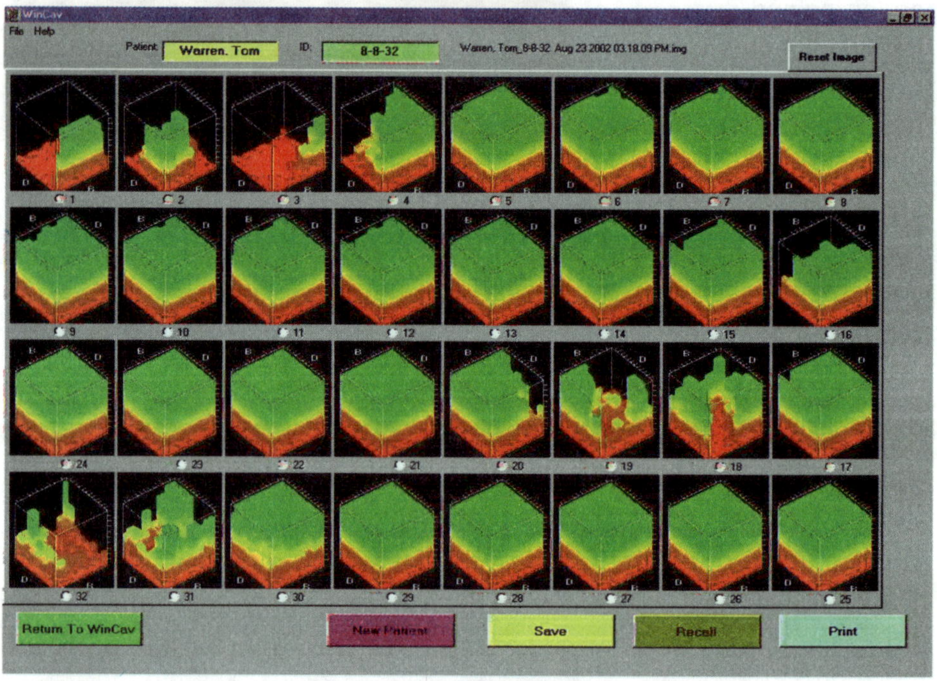

50 CAVITAT Medical Technologies (303) 755-2688.

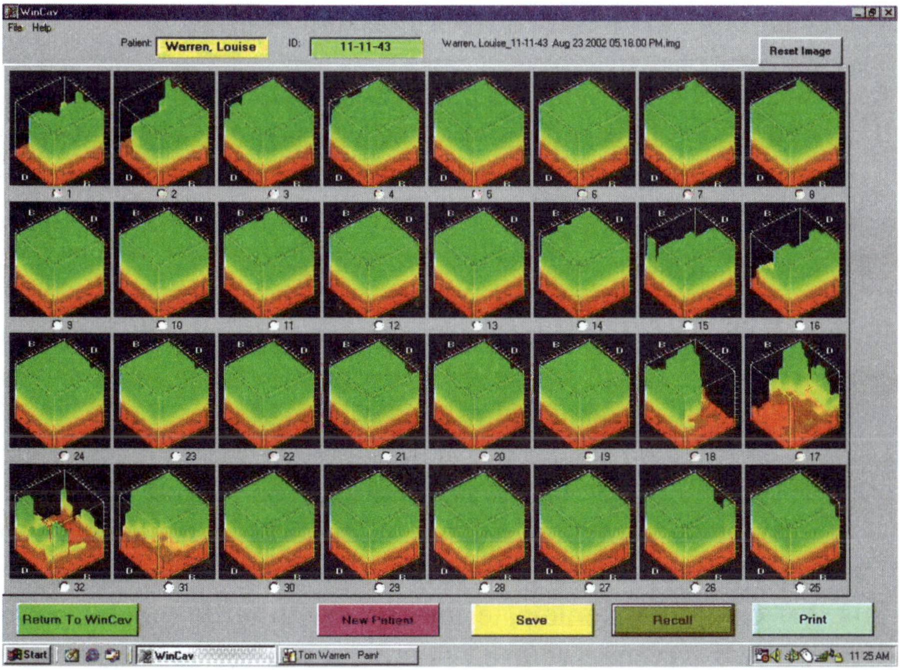

provides a 3-D image of the interior of the jawbone of suspected osteomyelitis (infection) sites. The Cavitat was designed for the needs of surgeons, who require a more accurate method to identify and accurately locate necrotic lesions.

Louise, my wife, appears healthy and seems free from outward signs of disease. Nonetheless, we are both going to have our jawbone infections taken care of immediately.

Dentists who use the Cavitat have taken more than 9,600 scans proven to be 97% accurate. Compare that figure to dental x-rays, which are 40% accurate. The Cavitat belongs in every dentist's office.

Looking At Mentally Ill Or Physically Sick People

1. 94% of all wisdom tooth sites are infected.

2. 96% of mouth areas where periodontal scaling has taken place are infected.

3. Cavitations can be caused from clots and bruises.

4. Most cavitations originate from root canals or sloppy dental housekeeping, e.g., the dentist does not completely clean up infection or thoroughly remove the infected periodontal ligament that attaches the tooth to the jawbone. All dry sockets will become infected. It is blood that causes regrowth of solid bone.

5. Introduction of streptococcus bacteria and closing off of oxygen as the bone heals causes aerobic bacteria to become anaerobic bacteria that will cause cavitations within 90 days.

Dentists normally use gutta percha to fill a drilled-out root canal. There is a relatively new product, calcium hydroxide, that prevents infection somewhat better than gutta percha, but there are no dental materials that completely eradicate infection within the tubules of root canals. It is the procedure itself that causes infectious organisms to proliferate. Over the last several years I have checked and rechecked this information with some of the most knowledgeable dental researchers and endodontists in the world who tell me root canals cannot be completely disinfected. Unfortunately, there is no such thing as a little infection. A little infection is like being a little pregnant.

Dr. Weston Price[51] demonstrated that by breaking off a small piece of a root-canalled tooth from a person who had died, let's say from heart disease, and implanting the fragment under the skin of a rabbit, the rabbit would die of heart disease. He re-implanted the same tooth under the skin of as many as 60 rabbits and they all died of heart disease within ten days. If the decedent had cancer of the liver, the rabbits all died from cancer of the liver. Whatever disease killed the patient killed the rabbits. If researchers implanted a piece of healthy tooth, the rabbit expelled the tooth through its skin, dissolved it, or

---

51 (1) *Dental Infections and Degenerative Diseases* (2) *Dental Infections: Oral and Systemic diseases* (3) *Nutrition and Physical Degeneration.* These books are available from the Price Pottenger Foundation (see references in Appendix X).

encapsulated the fragment within a protein shell and lived a normal life span. At the time of this research, the missing piece of the puzzle that could not be identified was how disease migrated from the jawbone throughout the body. Dentists and endodontists who did root canals spurned Dr. Price's research. In the early 1940s, penicillin was discovered and everyone assumed penicillin would kill infection in root canals and in the jawbone. It does not. According to Medline I and MEDLINE II,[52] there are 1,462-plus research papers from 1966 through July of 1997 linking infected teeth to focal infection.

A family member of a prominent scientist developed schizophrenia after getting one root canal. The gentleman heard enough about root canals to have the tooth extracted and the patient quickly recovered. This story is not an isolated incident. See Chapter 4.

Dr. Thomas Levy, who co-authored the book, *Uninformed Consent*, with Dr. Hal Huggins, told me he would rather have a whole mouthful of amalgam fillings than one root canal.

There are dentists who claim they can safely do root canals. They are not being honest with themselves or their patients. I know people with many root canals who close their minds to the science because of vanity, and consequently are suffering devastating diseases from schizophrenia, leukemia and cancer right next to the jawbone. They do not want false teeth.

What this boils down to is: the Cavitat accurately proves at least 95% of root canals become infected within 90 days. Expect the ADA and the American Association of Endodontists to do everything within their power to prevent news about the Cavitat from reaching the general public, because it will put root canal specialists out of business. The dental patients endodontists have injured and their attorneys can be expected to clean the cash out of endodontists' pockets and suck

---

52 MEDLINE is an Internet site providing access to medical abstracts from a database of over nine million citations. Pubmed.com offers this service free at http://www.ncbi.nlm.nih.gov/PubMed/.

up their insurance companies' reserves faster than a slick pickpocket.

Endodontists are considered the best mechanics in the dental industry. Purchase the Cavitat. It is the only instrument that gives the oral surgeon a clear view of diseased jawbone and educates the public about the menace of infectious diseases generated from root canals and jawbone infection. Everybody wins! The dentist saves the patient's health. Endodontists will make a good living as oral surgeons and earn their patients' respect and gratitude. That's one side of the coin.

What do you think is going to happen after it becomes common knowledge that our dentists have put their pocketbooks ahead of their patients' health? If endodontists continue to conceal the root canal issue like the ADA has stonewalled the fact that they have poisoned over 200 million Americans and had the arrogance to cover it up, endodontists should not expect to walk away with their money, or their reputations. Straighten this mess up before the public winds up despising you, before you become pariahs in our society.

What sick people really want to know is how to get well again, so let's cut to the chase!

Face Reality

There will never be a more important time to face what one must do to recover than there is right now. If you can't make yourself get off your duff and start walking,[53] if you care more about short-term rewards of stuffing yourself with junk food, soda pop, donuts and ice cream and lying around the house feeling like you've been beat up by Joe Louis than paying the price it takes to regain your thought process, go visit an Alzheimer's ward at your state mental hospital. If seeing the end stages of Alzheimer's disease does not motivate you to

53 Do not walk near traffic. For months I had to walk in the middle of the night to avoid auto exhaust fumes.

get on with life, throw this book in the garbage. No matter how much loved ones or your doctors want to help you recover, you are the one who must take action. You are in charge of your own destiny. The buck stops with you! In the beginning, when you are so exhausted it is easier to die than live, physical activity is more difficult than Army boot camp. But do it anyway. It gets easier. Later on, well, that's another story.

Later

Miracles do happen and when that day comes, the day you recognize that you are well again, your value system will change in an instant and the baggage you have shouldered for a lifetime will fall away faster than a rocket heading down range from Cape Canaveral. In a way that I do not seem able to express adequately, it is like being reborn. I carried so many misperceptions, anger and guilt for so many sins that it is amazing that I was able to stand up. The only reason the Lord Jesus bothered to save an old reprobate like me was to give me a chance to write this manuscript. He does not want His people to suffer such devastating diseases. I hope writing this book pleases the Lord and that some day, others might forgive the pain and trouble I caused in their lives.

Chapter 3

Getting Well Again

The separate treatments it takes to recover from mercurial poisoning are not difficult to learn by someone who is thinking clearly, but the patient's thought process, energy and will to survive are impaired. To make matters worse, people who have heavy metal poisoning often become obnoxious and difficult to work with. If that happens, caregivers need to keep this thought in mind. Remember how they used to be—they will become their old selves again.

If you are reading this book, either you, or someone you love, most likely has a serious medical condition that will destroy the patient unless they immediately begin to undertake the necessary actions to reverse the disease process. Over the years too many people bothered me time and again, claiming they wanted to get well, whose bottom line was: "I want to get well—if I don't have to do anything." They refused to take responsibility for their own life.

Are you willing to pay the price it takes to recover?

If you smoke, are a drug addict, an alcoholic or drink caffeinated beverages, eat a junk-food diet, consume sugar or substitute sugar in any form and continue to lead a hectic lifestyle, of if you have a petrochemical heating system and are unwilling to move, I am sorry—but unless you are willing to give all that up, don't bother to read any further; you'd be wasting your time. On the other hand, if there is something in your life more important than you, something worth paying the price it takes to recover, this section will be invaluable. At the end of this chapter you will find a summary of the procedures that I would use to reverse Alzheimer's disease under the heading, How To Get Well Again.

The Fly in the Ointment

Poisoned dental patients often develop a muddled thought process and a contentious personality. After they learn that they have iatrogenic disease[54], their confidence in the whole health-care profession evaporates. I have observed foggy, irritated, neurotic and sometimes-lazy patients with unrealistic expectations who complain because their dentist could not hand them a 15-cent magic bullet to cure their malady and allow them to continue living unhealthy lifestyles. Three of the most knowledgeable and caring dentists I know have quit clinical practice because of the hassle of dealing with dental boards, neurotic patients and frivolous lawsuits.

Caution

Medical professionals who know me personally have my unlisted telephone number. They will not mind if you verify our relationship. Along this same line, traditional family dentists have told really smart but gullible dental patients that "silver" amalgam does not contain mercury anymore. Ask them to put it in writing. Of course, they will not do that because they know you would sue them—because it does. Fifty percent of a silver amalgam dental filling is mercury.

Unrealistic Expectations

Most chronically ill patients who seek alternative treatments have seen many mainstream medical doctors who were unable to relieve their distress. Sometimes alternative practitioners are reluctant to ac-

---

54 Disease caused by inappropriate medical or dental treatment.

cept new patients who have been written off by their physicians, even if they think the patient has a reasonable chance of recovery, because if the patient dies, surviving spouses, relatives, attorneys, state dental and medical boards make more trouble than most alternative practice physicians care to deal with. A chiropractor told me about a woman near death who made a remarkable recovery only to focus on the fact she still had slight pain in one of her legs. Sooner or later every medical practitioner is going to have someone dissatisfied with the treatment process. Alternative caregivers are especially vulnerable because the establishment is frequently after their license. And, no matter how knowledgeable and vigilant a physician is, not everyone recovers.

How to begin the recovery process? Read!

Learn as much as you can. Knowing what to do will save you a small fortune in wasted medical expense and put you in charge of your own recovery program. This is crucial! Before anyone with brain-fog attempts to read new printed material, fan open the pages and dry the book out in the air for a week or two. With the exception of this book, new books usually out-gas formaldehyde fumes from glue that binds the manuscript to the spine, petrochemicals from ink that out-gas mercury and trace amounts of cyanide, and the paper is bleached white with chlorine.[55]

Reread this chapter, "Getting Well Again," until the pages fall apart. It is the simplest, easiest and least expensive way I can think of to learn what one must do to recover. Eventually you will realize that

---

55 Some environmental allergy patients are so sensitive to out-gassing petroleum fumes they live like hermits in the mountains and stow printed mail in garbage cans outside the house. All of these unfortunate people are low on trace minerals. I had to take trace minerals every day for more than four months before there was any noticeable improvement to cerebral brain-fog reactions from auto exhaust. Within 12 months most of the side effects from noxious smells abated.

every time you get in trouble you skipped something that did not seem important to you at the time. There are causes of short-term memory loss other than chronic low-level mercurial poisoning, root canal and jawbone infection, but the key to unlocking dozens of chronic diseases is getting rid of every:

- Mercury amalgam dental filling
- All of your root canals
- Every amalgam fragment in your gum tissue and jawbone and cleaning up jawbone infection (cavitations)

Finding the Right Dentist

Besides the patient's tenacity to stay the course, finding a really good dentist is the single most important step to recovery. All else in the treatment process hinges on his or her expertise. Be careful to find a dentist who has the specialized training to do the job right. They are few and far between. Fortunately, it is starting to be somewhat easier to find a well-trained physician and dentist who know how to treat chronic low-level mercurial poisoning now. More dentists, physicians and scientists have become aware of the mercury issue.

Remember this: There is a report from *Amalgam og Skydom* (*Dental Amalgam and Disease*) Oslo, Norway, 1993, by Dr. Harald J. Hamre that states, "If the patient is seriously ill, they are strongly advised against removing more than one or two small fillings at a time, with an interval of four to six weeks between amalgam removal sessions. Removing all amalgam in a very short time is well tolerated by most healthy people, but has repeatedly led to devastating long-lasting or even permanent disease in sensitive individuals."

The most logical approach to dental treatment is: no tooth, not the last tooth in your mouth, is worth saving if it damages your immune system. If the patient is seriously ill, there is a very narrow margin for error in removing and replacing mercury amalgam fillings. Most mercury-free dentists have specialized training to reduce the chances of permanent disability. It is the patient's pocketbook that pays the bill and it is the patient who will suffer the consequences of iatrogenic disease. If there was ever a time for the patient to take charge of his or her own recovery program, this is it!

Following is a list of questions to ask a potential dentist. If the patient is seriously ill, and the dental office cannot answer these questions correctly, leave. Find another dentist. Some dentists claim they can safely place root canals. It simply isn't true. Read Chapter 2 again. If I had any chronic disease of unknown origin, especially mental problems or any form of cancer, I would get rid of every root canal and cavitation in my mouth as well as every mercury amalgam filling, down to the smallest tattoo[56] and amalgam fragment within my gums and in the jawbone. I would insist on a biocompatibility blood test before allowing any—I mean any—dental materials to be inserted into my mouth.

56 A pool of mercury is often embedded in soft tissue of the oral cavity generated by an electrolysis reaction between gold crowns and a mercury filling in close proximity to one another

Ask the dentist	The Answer Should Be
Does he place mercury-amalgam fillings? If a dentist still continues to place mercury fillings, a patient exhibiting signs of chronic disease should not even be in his office. It is contaminated with mercury. Leave.	No
Does he do root canals?	No
Does he remove amalgam fragments and tattoos?	Yes
Does he treat cavitations or can he refer you to a surgeon who does?	Yes
Does he do materials biocompatibility testing?	Yes
Does he make consecutive 7-day appointments?	No

Dentists who ignore materials biocompatibility testing do not realize that after a person's immune system has been compromised, they are treating a patient who can be allergic to almost anything. Everybody's different. If you have neurological, mental disease or cancers, do not skip the biocompatibility blood test.

"Do not allow your dentist to use any materials that have not been approved. What is safe for your brother, your sister, or father and mother and a hundred thousand other dental patients might be your undoing."

—Dr. Huggins

Getting What You Pay For

The only thing that belongs in anyone's mouth is his or her own teeth, or biocompatible dental materials, period. If you cannot think clearly, or if you are not feeling well, you will be unable to help yourself recover. This is serious business. Don't jump from the frying pan into the fire. Do it right or don't do it at all. Your dentist is not in charge here. You are! It's your pocketbook that pays his bill. If the dentist wants to skip a few things. Fire him! Get out of his chair and find another dentist. Referrals to biocompatibility testing facilities and well-trained mercury-free dentists will be found in Appendix IX.

Dr. Huggins tells me the safest filling material available is 82% 24-karat gold and 18% platinum, Unfortunately, 3% of the population are allergic to gold and 1% are allergic to platinum. There are more than 1750 chemicals and filling materials available to dentists, and the chances of randomly selecting totally safe biocompatible materials that dental patients suffering from chronic disease will not have problems with are about the same as winning the Lotto. To reiterate: If you have chronic disease, before you have any work done by a dentist, get a materials biocompatibility blood test. In addition, the same test will determine the correct vitamins, minerals, hormones and enzymes needed for healing to occur. The patient will require nutritional and/or hormonal supplements before, during, and after amalgam removal. See Appendix II. The good thing about doing all this is that within six months, provided your fillings were correctly removed, jawbone infection cleaned up, you continue walking two miles three times a week and lead a healthy lifestyle, you'll be well along the road to recovery.

In the meantime realize that with one exception, psychologists who treat neurosis (mixed-up thought process), no neurologist or psychiatrist who uses psychotropic medications to control his or her patient's behavior, gene-splicing specialist or any other physician is likely to permanently cure the mental and neurological diseases referred to in this book until the smallest fragment of mercury is removed from the patient's teeth, jawbone and gums and all the patient's root canals have been "properly"[57] removed, which means the periodontal ligament needs to be excised deeper than most dentists realize, about one millimeter deeper, to prevent jawbone reinfection.

Kinesiology

Most people who have chronic disease lose their earning capacity. For those with modest means who cannot afford biocompatible blood tests, the kinesiology test is the best alternative.

Provided I was able to scrape up a couple of hundred dollars, I'd prefer the biocompatibility blood test. I'd rather have all my teeth pulled than risk another wad of dough on incompatible dental materials. Been there. Done that—twice. An actor, whose name almost everyone in the United States would recognize, had to have $30,000[58] worth of dental work replaced within three weeks because he reacted to the new dental materials in his mouth.

Getting back to kinesiology, this is how it works: the dentist will put a dental material he plans to test in one of the patient's hands and ask the patient to extend his or her opposite arm. He will face his patient squarely, not smile or frown, and place one of his hands on the patient's shoulder. He will press on the patient's extended arm that will either lock in place or drop. It does not take much pressure. If the patient is allergic to a specific substance, the dentist should be able to push a piano mover's arm down with two fingers. If the substance is biocompatible, the patient's arm will lock in place. For testing nutritional supplements, hold an unopened bottle of a specific vitamin in the hand before making the purchase and do this same test. It does not

---

57 This is not amateur night. If you are seriously ill and have been going to a mainstream ADA dentist, you're not only in the wrong church; you're sitting in the wrong pew. Make sure the dentist you go to has not been placing silver fillings for many years.

58 In 2002 dollars the $30,000 figure would be approximately $100,000.

always work, but it has saved me a great deal of money.

Electrical Tests

Physicians who understand the body's electrical system sometimes use a Dermatron machine, an electrical device, to test how specific vitamins and dental materials affect the body's energy at acupuncture meridians. It is extremely accurate. The only drawback is that it is too time-consuming to be cost-effective. In addition, doctors like to see the physical evidence for themselves that blood tests reveal.

The Food Allergy Chemical Sensitivity Connection to Chronic Disease

It is unlikely the patient, their family physician, psychiatrist or neurologist will suspect a chemical sensitivity or food allergy connection to mental or chronic disease. Remember that allergies are not the underlying cause of the patient's illness; they are a symptom of a weakened immune system that is more often than not caused by mercury amalgam dental fillings, root canals, jawbone infection and malnutrition.

Decontaminate Your Living Area

A young woman moved into an apartment that had been heavily sprayed with insecticide to eradicate cockroaches. She became deathly ill. For many years I allowed thousands of people to call me for information, until the pressure and expense of working one-on-one became unbearable. This young woman's constant calling bordered on harassment and was one of the reasons we moved and changed to an unlisted telephone number many times before life began to return to normal. I told her repeatedly to clean up the newspapers she had strewn upon the floor of her apartment, then to move into an uncontaminated building with baseboard electric heat. She was exhausted and over the period of the six months that she telephoned had not picked up the newspapers, cleaned anything or moved. The woman called me one last time with the same complaints, etc. This was the only time this happened, but I blew my cork and screamed, "Clean up the place! Move, or die! Don't bother me anymore!" A half-year or so later I was talking with a friend when a lovely young woman interrupted our conversation saying, "You don't know me, do you?" She was obviously quite well, almost radiant. The woman had moved and had her mercury fillings replaced.

The Clean Room

My wife and I had previously purchased attractive cotton materials to reupholster several chairs from a company that was going out of business. The upholstery business we chose to recover our furniture had a reputation for doing the highest-quality work in town. Even so, their showroom reeked from formaldehyde fumes out-gassing from hundreds of bolts of synthetic materials they used in their business, and it was obvious that the owner was chemically sensitive. It turned out that she had purchased *Beating Alzheimer's* three years before but had not bothered to read it. So I told her either I know what I'm talking about or I don't, and you can determine the truth for yourself about that in 24 hours for less than 200 dollars.[59] And she did. The next day she was radiant. She took four of her friends to breakfast the following morning to tell them how wonderful she felt.

This is what I told her to do:

Make an Oasis

Purchase two plain white 100 percent cotton sheets, two cotton pillowcases, two heavy large white beach towels of 100 percent cotton

---

59 That was roughly ten years ago. The two-hundred-dollar figure would be closer to four hundred dollars.

and two cotton bath towels, two 100 percent cotton blankets and two new pillows made from quallofill that does not out-gas odors. If you already have plain white 100 percent cotton sheets, pillowcases, towels and blankets, use them, but wash them according to the following instructions. The pillows need to be new, however. Also buy "unscented" laundry soap to wash everything. Use about one half of the amount of laundry soap as would normally be necessary. Rinse twice. Dr. Randolph told me cotton is one of the most heavily chemicalized crops in the United States. So, if this effort is to have value, rinse everything, twice.

Hopefully the room you chose for a clean room will be a bedroom that has a very clean, old carpet—or, better yet, a wood floor—and hopefully your home uses an electric heating system. In any case, for this test, close the air vents in the bathroom and bedroom and cover the air vents with aluminum foil and duct-tape the edges so that air from the rest of the living quarters does not contaminate the clean room. It is particularly important to seal the vents and to shut the bedroom door if the home has a wood, coal or any sort of petrochemical heating system.

If the bedroom adjoins the bathroom, remove every scented object, including soap from the bathroom and everything from under the sink. Stow those items in some other room.

Buy a can of Bon Ami® scouring powder to clean the bathroom shower and sink. Throw all your chlorinated scouring powders in the garbage. Purchase unscented shampoo and a bar of unscented hand soap. If your water contains chlorine, close the bathroom door and do not open it during the night. Use another bathroom.

Strip everything out of the bedroom except an old-fashioned wind-up metal clock. This includes the bed—mattresses are full of chemicals, dust mites and other cooties. For a couple of nights you will have to sleep on the floor.

Totally clean everything out of the closet. Closets tend to collect dust and mold. In addition, everybody has some synthetic clothing in the closet and no matter how lovely synthetic clothing appears, if you want to get well again, give all of that stuff away. Sounds absurd, doesn't it? When this test is over, you will feel like throwing the whole kit and caboodle on the floor and stomping all over it. If you are not allergic to wool, cotton and wool are the materials of choice.

Dust the tops of doorjambs and any other place dust accumulates with a slightly damp cloth. Very carefully vacuum the bedroom carpet and/or damp-mop a wooden floor and rinse it with clear water. Preferably use a water vacuum, because regular vacuum cleaners leave fine dust particles in the air. If you do not have a water vac, vacuum the carpet, change your vacuum cleaner bag and do it over again.

Provided the bedroom windows do not face the street and there are no scented flowers, trees or shrubs in the yard, and provided the prevailing wind from a factory or busy street does not blow toward the window, open the bedroom window 1/4 inch and shut the bedroom door. Closing all the bedroom doors cuts off the air supply to the clean room; you need to open the window 1/4 inch to provide enough oxygen to breathe throughout the night.

Lay a cotton sheet over two cotton towels on the carpet, and/or on a cotton blanket if you need the comfort. Cover yourself with a cotton sheet and cotton blankets.[61]

Some discount stores sell "odiferous" feather blankets and pillows. Do not buy them. Never use feather pillows. Not only are they a waste of money, feather pillows and dust mites cause sensitive people brain-

---

61 Louise sews two white cotton sheets together to make blanket covers for our goose down comforters. I am slightly allergic to goose down, but as long as I keep the cotton slipcover over the blanket, there does not seem to be a problem.

fog. Throw out your pillows once or twice a year. (Quallofill pillows do not out-gas detectable chemicals and are inexpensive.) After two years, 25 percent of the weight of a pillow is dust mites. There is a story about old pillows causing brain-fog in *Beating Alzheimer's*.

In a clear glass, porcelain or a high-grade stainless-steel pot, boil enough hot water to drink in the morning. Heating water releases chlorine. Never use an aluminum container.

Before you retire, take a shower and wash your hair with unscented shampoo, and use unscented soap on the rest of your body. It might not be a good idea to snuggle up for any length of time, because you will be breathing out-gassing mercury vapor from your spouse's dental fillings.

That's all. That's the test. How did you feel when you woke up? Is your head clear? Later in the day, as you contact favorite foods and environmental chemicals, you will begin to feel hung over. Don't worry, because you're going to fix the problem. It takes a little work, but brain-fog will eventually disappear, you will regain your strength and your life will (almost) return to normal.

Do not shower in the morning. Chlorinated water from washing your face or shaving is enough of a problem. In due course, you will purchase a whole house water filter to remove chlorine from the drinking water, showers, washing machine and toilets.

Caution: Whatever else you do, do not use scented cleansers or hair spray when you clean up in the morning. Perfume and hair spray are loaded with chemicals that provoke brain-fog and will cause you to feel like taking a long walk on a short pier. Throw all your perfume and hair spray in the trashcan. Stay away from anyone who uses hair spray, perfume, shaving lotion or noxious-smelling under-arm deodorants. That is the reason to shower before going to bed: to wash the chemicals away.

If you still do not feel well the next morning, tear out the bedroom carpet and get rid of it. If a carpet is less than seven years old,[62] it still contains formaldehyde. If necessary, remove pressed board sub-flooring and install a wood, tile, or slate floor. Wash the walls if you want, but do not repaint the clean room. Or in the summertime, open the windows and dry the paint out for 30 days before people who exhibit symptoms of brain-fog sleep there.[63] The only wood sealer I was able to tolerate was Swedish Finish that really "stinks" until it dries for three or four days.[64] Swedish Finish dries so hard it barely out-gases odor. Given my druthers, I'd choose Swedish Finish, because it is easier to maintain than bee's wax. Bee's wax is the only preservative that I know to be completely safe for chemically sensitive brain-allergy sufferers.

Presuming you passed the cotton test the first night, the second night bring clean wool blankets into the clean room. If wool is okay, bring the mattress and bed back the third night. But throw the mattress pad in the garbage. The shells of mattress pads are loaded with formaldehyde. Put two washed, woolen or cotton blankets on the mattress (they must not be odiferous)[65], and place two large white 100-percent cotton towels on the blankets and a 100-percent cotton sheet over the towels. This is necessary because chemically sensitive brain-allergy

---

62 Multi-colored carpets contain formaldehyde for ten years.

63 The same results can be obtained by closing the bedroom door, opening a window about 1/4 inch and turning up the heat to 75 degrees for a week.

64 Open the clean room window and seal off that part of the house for three or four days with plastic. It is worth the effort. I had a wooden floor installed in our bedroom (clean room).

65 We purchased two wool blankets from an army surplus store that I had to wash four times in a Laundromat's oversized commercial washing machine, because they were loaded with mothball fumes. We dried them slowly on "low heat"for quite a while before they dried. We put two large white 100% cotton beach towels over the wool blankets, one for Louise and another for myself, and two heavy cotton towels over the cotton beach towels and a cotton fitted sheet over everything. We change the top sheet and first layer of cotton towels once a week. About every two weeks, we wash all the towels on the bed. Probably

sufferers react to synthetic materials used in mattresses. You need a barrier between the mattress and you. Never use scented laundry soap. Give all of your scented soap away.

The first night, it is all right to hang washed 100-percent cotton clothing in the closet. If you had no reaction to this, the next night bring in clean 100-percent wool clothing that has never been dry-cleaned. Last, bring in woolen clothing that has been dry-cleaned. You will quickly learn which items to avoid.

Do not use electric blankets. Electricity stresses the immune system and the chemical fumes out-gassing from insulation on electrical wiring often provoke brain-fog in chemically sensitive allergy patients or may exacerbate some other medical problem.

Sooner than later, the patient is going to become spaced out and feel miserable from food allergy or environmental chemicals that they inadvertently expose themselves to. The clean room provides a relatively uncontaminated environment to crash until brain-fog clears. It is impossible to recover without making a clean room.

The Mercury Allergy Chain of Events

Mercury poisons the brain and disassembles the myelin sheath surrounding the synapse, causing neuronal death and the neurofibillary tangles which pathologists see in Alzheimer's diseased brain tissue. In addition, mercury binds to the oxygen-carrying sites on red blood cells. Oxygen gets off wherever it is needed, while mercury binds to the hemoglobin until the cell dies, which makes the body produce additional red blood cells to supply the brain with enough oxygen to

---

every six months, sometimes longer, we go to the laundromat to wash the woolen army blankets. I learned this from Dr. Randolph. All of his allergy patients follow this procedure. Do not use scented laundry soap.

survive. Mercury also penetrates the heart and intestinal walls, the kidneys,[66] the arteries within the brain, and causes arteriosclerosis in the heart, the arteries in our necks, and even in the veins in our ankles, causing our heart to work harder.

All of the mercury toxic patients Dr. Huggins tested had low hydrochloric stomach acid, a condition that allows candida to proliferate. Both mercury and candida bore through the intestines into the blood stream, causing candida to become systemic.[67] In addition, low stomach acid causes food to putrefy, further damaging the intestinal wall allowing undigested protein to pass into the bloodstream. The body does not recognize putrefied protein as nutrition and develops antibodies causing brain allergy against that specific food. In addition, flukes, fungus and parasites pass through the leaky colon to set up housekeeping in other parts of the body. The brain cannot get enough blood, oxygen or nutrition, causing it to starve to death. Very simply: the cure for dozens of chronic diseases is reversing all of those symptoms. First: let's clear up your thought process and restore your energy.

Allergies

Allergies are the sign of a stressed immune system. In the beginning, cerebral allergy sufferers tend to develop such mild allergies that they shrug them off before they begin to recognize specific symptoms of disease. If you notice a slight reaction to pollens or dust, you are also allergic to favorite foods, molds, metals, and chemicals—almost anything. There is no such thing as one allergy.

---

66 The kidneys retain more mercury than any other organ in the body.
67 Pertaining to, or afflicting the body as a whole.

The Provocative Challenge Test

1.

Write down your ten favorite foods on a stenography pad (that has a line down the middle of the page). Keep the steno pad as your record. Months, even 20 years later, when the allergy sufferer does not feel well, he or she will have inadvertently consumed a food or come in contact with an environmental chemical that provokes the identical cerebral or physical reaction as the original test.

2.

When you wake up in the morning, sit on the side of the bed and take your pulse. Write it down on the left-hand side of the page. Write the time down too. Before breakfast, sit down and take your pulse again. Write down your pulse rate and the time again on the left.

3.

On the right side of the steno book, write down how you feel.

4.

Eat an ordinary breakfast. It should contain only one of the favorite foods on your list.

5.

Write down every scrap of food or drink you consumed for breakfast on the left side of the page. If you feel miserable any time during the day, write down the time and your reaction on the right side of the page. You may or may not be able to write well. Writing is a cerebral motor function. When your head is clear, you may have beautiful handwriting. If you have brain allergy and are allergic to a specific food or drink, or come in contact with some other toxic environmental chemical, your handwriting will deteriorate.

6.

For this test (do not read books or newspapers) quietly take your pulse at 15-minute intervals for one hour. If your pulse has risen eight or more points, you are allergic to something you ate for breakfast.

7.

In that case, at the next meal eat as much as you want of any one food on your list of foods you ate at breakfast. If your pulse does not rise eight points and your handwriting is normal an hour after eating this particular food, in all probability you are not allergic to that specific food. If you suspect the food might be a problem anyway, repeat the identical test for dinner. If there is no reaction, it is a safe food. Allergy-free foods are like having money in the bank. Keep on testing the original breakfast foods, only one food at each meal, until you have tested every food you had for breakfast the first day. Remember, I am talking about three meals a day. If you had toast, butter and strawberry jam for breakfast, you will need to check toast by itself, butter (substitute milk for butter) by itself, and strawberry jam by itself. Be sure to use the identical bread, butter (milk) and jam as in your first test, because different brands of foods sometimes use unique chemicals and dissimilar ingredients. One bread in particular gives me a pounding headache right between my eyes. Another bakery produces a similar product, but does not use monosodium glutamate (MSG). Their bread does not cause a headache or brain-fog. As you eliminate or learn to rotate foods in your diet that you are sensitive to, your pulse rate will steadily decline to normal levels.

8.

Try to rotate your foods over a four-day period. It takes, on average, four days for food to pass completely through your alimentary canal. If you do not rotate foods, at least make an effort to expand the variety of your diet and do not eat wheat, corn or drink milk every day. If you have food allergies and continually consume the same food, eventually it will produce allergic reactions, causing cerebral allergy brain-fog, brain-fag, or physical symptoms of disease.

Pollen Allergies

Luckily, pollen allergies are easy to reverse. Wherever you live, in the coldest part of the year, find a beekeeper in your area who will sell you honeycomb. This is one case in which more is not better, more antidotes the remedy.[69] Consume only a one-inch thin slice of honeycomb once each month for three months. Chew it until every bit of the honeycomb is dissolved. Take trace minerals every other day and forget about pollen allergy until the following year. It is a good idea to clear away scotch broom and odiferous trees surrounding your immediate living area. Whatever you do, do not use chemicals to eradicate them. Purchase a dust respirator from Mine Safety Appliances, whose telephone number is 1 (800) MSA-2222 anywhere in the United States. You may need to move to the seashore on the West Coast where the prevailing wind blows east from the Pacific Ocean. Make sure the heating system you choose is electric. Do not use a wood stove, fireplace or petrochemical heating system.

Other Chemical Sensitivities

My mother was a dental assistant and suffered from schizophrenia most of her life. After I learned about the mercury/cerebral allergy connection to mental disease, it was easy to understand the underlying cause of her distress and bizarre behavior. Psychiatrists do not understand the allergy/chemical sensitivity connection to depression, schizophrenia, or Alzheimer's, much less the patient's need for vitamin and mineral supplementation. If you or a loved one has mental problems, find an orthomolecular psychiatrist.

I can tell you who does know: NASA executives, submarine com-

69 Homeopathic remedies are diluted poisons, which provoke the identical reaction in healthy people as found in a specific disease. As the body cures the reaction to the homeopathic remedy, it cures the disease.

manders and insurance adjusters.[70] They do not have the whole picture, but they know more about the underlying cause of inexplicably bizarre behavior than anyone except environmental allergists. Servicemen with long and distinguished careers have become disoriented and developed hallucinations after being exposed to out-gassing paint fumes in submarines.[71]

Government environmental physicians found the peace lily and the spider plant are particularly hearty and that they absorb toxic fumes like a vacuum cleaner. In warmer climates, the Chinese evergreen works well but is not as hearty as the peace lily (important: always cut buds off indoor plants to minimize pollen in the air from blooms). To give you an example, as a test, I purchased a table made from pressed wood that reeked of formaldehyde, a leather chair loaded with mercury residue and a bookcase that smelled horrible from formaldehyde fumes. There are a couple of hundred books on my shelves out-gassing petrochemical fumes, formaldehyde, mercury, trace amounts of cyanide and other chemicals within five feet of my work station. I also have two very large healthy peace lilies several feet from my chair and plan to purchase a spider plant. In addition, our condominium has an air exchanger constantly circulating outside air throughout the structure. Ninety percent of the inside air is exchanged once every hour. It took me years to learn how to protect myself. There are many other things to learn before attempting to duplicate the above scenario. Do not attempt to make such a foolish purchase of toxic furniture until you really know how to protect yourself. The primary reason I purchased these noxious furnishings was to test for brain-fog reactions to these odiferous products before we published this book, and I can say for certain that if the peace lilies were not adequately cleaning up my office, I would have set the furniture out in a vented

70 Insurance adjusters know because they pay the claims and evoke a confidentiality clause in the contract to prevent the injured party from informing the public about the incident.

71 Chemists eventually learned how to decontaminate the paint.

storage shed for a year or returned it to the store and boxed every book in the office and put them outside in the garage.

Environmental Chemicals

The reason chemically sensitive people need to avoid hydrocarbon fumes in fossil fuels, especially from diesel exhaust and coal, is because petrochemical fumes out-gas trace amounts of mercury vapor and cyanide. In addition, wood, coal, gas, oil, butane heating systems and candles consume oxygen. Candlewicks out-gas lead. Newsprint out-gases petrochemical fumes. Out-gassing hydrocarbons from newsprint can cause a chemically sensitive person to become spaced out in two seconds. I know of only one woman who suffered from short-term memory loss who continued using a fossil-fuel heating system (gas) who has completely recovered.

We recently moved to a high ridge overlooking a spectacular panoramic view of the Cascade Mountains. The builders used special ties to keep the roof from blowing off during windstorms. Speaking for myself, I love the wind. It cleans the air. Our condominium has a gas furnace and I had made up my mind to tear it out and install an electric furnace before we moved in. It turned out that the builders also installed an air exchanger. With the exception of very expensive homes built by the area's foremost builders, every other home I have ever been in outgases chemical residue from new construction materials and gas furnaces. However, there was no odor in our condo that I noticed except when painters touched up several holidays on the walls (thin paint spots painters sometimes miss during construction). The next day, paint smell was so obnoxious we came within a half inch of walking away from our earnest money to find an older home. Luckily, we waited a few days to recheck chemical contamination and the odors had evaporated. Our unit had a clean smell again. The furnace room also has a recirculation system and, except for a brief time when I turned on the gas hot-water heater in the furnace room, I have not noticed gas fumes any place in the home. More importantly, my eyes do not exhibit the ubiquitous shiners[72] that chemically sensitive patients exhibit when they are exposed to hydrocarbon fumes. All people who are allergic to hydrocarbon fumes have low trace mineral levels. We'll get to the remedy later.

Formaldehyde and Toxic Chemicals

Formaldehyde is one of the most common indoor pollutants, is listed by National Toxicology Program (NTP) and International Agency for Research on Cancer (ARC) and regulated by Occupational Safety and Health Administration (OSHA) as a potential carcinogen. The literature indicates teachers and students who handle preserved specimens represent potential high-exposure groups. Most of us are exposed to formaldehyde fumes through its use in new construction materials, pressed wood products, textiles, home furnishings, paper and cosmetics. At particularly high risk for formaldehyde exposure are residents of mobile homes containing particleboard and plywood and persons living in conventional homes insulated with urea-formaldehyde foam. Attention Deficit Disorder (ADD), brain-fog and brain-fag can be triggered by out-gassing toxic chemicals from new construction, carpets, cleaning compounds—floor wax used in older schools on wooden floors—by formaldehyde, hydrocarbon and chlorine fumes from new books and mold from old books. Teachers can determine if a child is chemically sensitive by opening a new book and putting it directly into the face of a student with ADD and asking the student to take a whiff. Do not make a big deal of it; just go about your teaching, but do

72 Chemically sensitive people who have out-gassing petrochemical, coal or wood heating systems or leave books and newspapers lying around tend to have dark circles under their eyes, causing one to think they spent an uneasy sleepless night. Sometimes that is the case. They just need more sleep. Most of the time it means changing your heating system to electricity, or better yet, move.

not be surprised if the student cannot keep his or her eyes open. To avoid these reactions, fan open the pages and air out schoolbooks for two weeks and notice the improvement in students' attention span and behavior. Better yet, insist that book manufacturers do not use petrochemical inks in schoolbooks. Vegetable dye is the ink of choice.

The first clues to cerebral allergic reactions in children are students who cannot keep their eyes open, can't sit still, the class cut-ups, stutterers or students who exhibit sloppy, scribbly, heavy or illegible handwriting. I remember a teacher yelling at me, "Hey spring fever, wake up!" Everyone had smiles on their faces. It was a beautiful spring day, the sun was warm, the windows were open, the pollens were out, and I had spring fever—and my nose in a new book. Spring fever is a distinct marker for pollen allergy.

This is not well known, but miniscule amounts of radiation, mercury, cadmium and lead that leach from television sets and computer monitors sometimes cause brain-fog and/or brain-fag in sensitive intervals. Read *The Impossible Child*, provided it is still available, otherwise, *Is This Your Child* by Dr. Doris Rapp. If the student has mercury amalgam fillings, have the school nurse check the student's symptoms against those in Appendix I. Flat computer screens do not cause brain-fog. The safest thing to do with old computer monitors is to dump them in the garbage.

The Problem with New Buildings

If new construction is not built too tightly, it takes about seven years for buildings to out-gas most of their toxic chemicals. Fifteen or so years ago, we lived near a lovely small town by the sea where well-to-do retired people built huge new homes along the seashore. The standard heating system was gas.[73] Shortly after they moved in, I noticed that an unusual number of our new neighbors became reclusive.

---

73 We had an electric baseboard heating system.

Oftentimes the scuttlebutt was that one or the other of the spouses had developed Alzheimer's. Alzheimer's disease might have been the official diagnosis, but in reality most of those people—probably all of them—had developed cerebral allergies[74] to out-gassing chemicals from gas furnaces, formaldehyde fumes from new carpets and other out-gassing chemicals in wallboard, glues and paint. Indoor air pollution can build up to be ten times higher in tight, new buildings than outside air. Revised building codes in King County, Washington, require air exchangers to be installed in new construction to reduce indoor air pollution.

Mercury was removed from indoor latex wall paint in August of 1990 and replaced with formaldehyde.[75] Both substances prevent mold. Toxic chemicals are a two-edged sword, because chemicals that retard mold, fungus and bacteria, and kill insects, have an accumulative toxic synergistic effect on all living tissue.[76] After our immune system has been compromised, people can become hypersensitive to minute amounts of chemicals, pollens and their favorite foods. They are "universal reactors" and living becomes more difficult than I can bear to remember. Many, perhaps most of these unfortunate people do not function well in society. They often become irritable, reclusive, depressed, paranoid, or develop schizophrenia. Many of them become alcoholics and/or drug addicts.

Our Farmland Is Poisoned

The chemical industry has been disposing of hazardous toxins they cannot economically get rid of by mixing the contaminants with fertilizer, and farmers have unintentionally spread toxic waste on the

---

74 Chemical sensitivity is a more accurate word than allergy.

75 Later on a physician retested indoor Latex wall paint for mercury contamination. Twenty-five percent of the formulas still contained mercury. Apparently all that some of the manufacturers did was change their labels.

land for years. It reminds me of the book entitled *Toxic Sludge Is Good For You*, by John C. Stauber and Sheldon Rampton. The Seattle Times newspaper exposed the chemical industry's scam in a series of stories by Duff Wilson[77] entitled "Fear In the Fields," in 1999. Instead of putting those responsible for the chicanery in the penitentiary, the Washington State legislature allowed the practice to continue, because giant grain producers whose incomes were affected by the revelations did their utmost to whitewash the issue for economic reasons. To sell contaminated grain and foodstuffs to the international market is an inexcusable breach of ethics. The only way this idiotic practice will stop is if foreign nations refuse to import Washington produce.

Water Filters

Industrial chemicals and farm animals pollute most all of the land and water in industrialized nations. American cities usually decontaminate drinking water with chlorine, and mercury is used in the manufacturing process of chlorine. Recovery is impossible if you expose yourself to chlorine. You will need to purchase a whole house water filter. See Appendix IX.

Outside of medical and dental expenses, converting to an electric heating system and installing a whole house water filtering system, and/or moving away from a highly contaminated environment are the most expensive costs of getting well again.

I recall a story by one of the members of the Well Mind Association.[78]

---

76 *Our Stolen Future*, Theo Colburn, Dianne Dumanoski and John Peterson Myers, Plume/Penguin.

77 Duff Wilson recently published a new book entitled *Fateful Harvest* that any nation contemplating purchasing Northwest grains and produce needs to read.

78 Well Mind Association, Seattle, Washington (206) 547-6167.

The woman told me she visited younger relatives (both physicians) several months earlier at their beautiful new home in another state. She said there was such intense hostility between the couple you could slice it with a knife. Shortly after my friend returned to Seattle, the couple separated and the demoralized husband took time off to recuperate at an older home along the Pacific Coast seashore. Four days later he felt relaxed and had regained the tranquility missing in his life. He telephoned his wife to come to the ocean and the same thing happened to her. They sold their new house, built another home from old materials, and became a happy loving family.

The reason the Alzheimer's patients recognize loved ones and seem relatively normal one day, then become hostile or do not know their own children on the next, is because of exposure to chemicals or food allergies that produce swelling in the brain.[79] Food allergy, pollen allergy, and chemical susceptibility are more intertwined with erratic behavior, schizophrenia and short-term memory loss than psychiatrists or neurologists realize. But again I repeat that cerebral allergies are not the underlying cause of Alzheimer's disease or schizophrenia. Mercury amalgam dental fillings and root canals are the primary problem. Mercury poisons the brain and weakens the immune system, opening the door to cerebral allergy and many, many other medical problems. Professor Mats Hansen, PhD, who led the Swedish amalgam war that caused politicians to discontinue the use of mercury fillings, writes that 208 diseases have been traced to mercury in silver amalgam dental fillings. I know Mats personally. He is among the smartest scientists, professors and doctors whom I know. If Mats writes mercury dental fillings cause 208 diseases, believe it.

Potency of Combinations of Toxic Substances

What the public needs to urgently recognize is that when a specific

79 There are several examples of these phenomena in my first book, *Beating Alzheimer's.*

poison is combined with any other toxin, you have a different, far more potent poison.

The Environmental Protection Agency says:

There are more than 70,000 untested chemicals used in the United States. If any combination of three (3) hazardous chemicals is taken into the body, the synergistic effect is 5,000 times more toxic than any one chemical by itself. [80]

One hundred percent of human fat tissue samples tested from nine regions in the United States contained chemicals including Styrene (found in Styrofoam), Dichlorobenzene (found in mothballs, household cleaners and deodorizers), Xylene or Benzene (found in paints and gasoline) and DDT that has been banned since 1972. These chemicals accumulate in the body's fat and tissue; they mimic hormones and create havoc with emotions and stamina, and destroy brain cells. The five most toxic trace metals found were lead, mercury, aluminum, cadmium and beryllium. These metals are suspected of being the origin of at least 50 percent of all premature deaths and of causing many other disabling diseases. To the furthermost islands, to the poles of the earth, human adipose tissue has accumulated on average more than 400 chemicals in body fat.

Dr. Theron Randolph, the world-renowned environmental allergist, told me 20 years ago that in three generations our entire population will become as ill as I was in 1982. The whole world ought to read my medical records. Thousands of species of wildlife are disappearing and human beings are at the top of the food chain. We breathe in and ingest more varieties of toxic substances than any other species. If we continue to remain ambivalent about getting rid of mercury amalgam

---

80 Environmental Protection Agency, *National Human Adipose Tissue Survey* FY82, 560/5-86-039, December 1986.

dental fillings and cleaning up our environment, the message in this book will be meaningless, because if Dr. Randolph's prediction is accurate, the human race will have become too ill and poor in two more generations to take remedial action to reverse human extinction.

By the time you recognize an odor, minute amounts of the out-gassing substance have passed from your lungs into your blood stream or from your nose to your brain. In addition, you lose approximately 50 percent of your ability to distinguish offending odors within 24 hours. In other words, if you remain in a contaminated building for 24 hours, your nose will have lost one half of its ability to protect you. The chemicals it cannot detect will still be doing their damage, but you will be unaware of their presence. The mental and physical repercussions from living or working in a chemically contaminated environment come on so subtly that most people—not even their family physician—will not have a clue to the origin of their distress. If you find yourself becoming edgy or irritable, if you are beginning to feel spacey and worn out, that is the time to seek an environmental physician and a mercury-free dentist. The new home and petrochemical heating system or newly painted walls are important clues. Dr. Randolph had his patients remove more than 3,000 wood, coal, gas stoves and other petrochemical heating systems from their homes. Not one patient ever complained.

Food Allergy

Most neurologists and psychiatrists seem unaware that food allergies and chemical susceptibilities are involved with schizophrenia or Alzheimer's disease. It doesn't fit their paradigm. As noted in Chapter 1, Dr. Fudenberg took an Alzheimer's patient who was flat on her back out of an Alzheimer's ward and restored her to vibrant health with a treatment protocol he calls the "Transfer Factor." The Transfer Factor transfers another healthy person's immunity to a chronically ill patient, allowing the patient to recover.

Food allergies are addictive. One side of the coin is allergies; the other side is addiction. Giving up coffee, cigarettes, alcohol and drugs will cause addicts to feel as if they have been run over by a loaded gravel truck. Abstaining from favorite foods causes similar temporary reactions for several days. It takes me about five and one-half days to clear. Then, I feel wonderful! If it were possible, I would never eat again.

I have given much thought to the food allergy[81] connection to cerebral allergies and chronic disease, because there is no easy solution to solve this problem. In his time, Dr. Randolph was the world's most informed physician about the realities of addictive food allergies. He developed a method to isolate foods and chemicals that provoke physical or mental symptoms of disease that he coined brain-fog and brain-fag. Brain-fog, if left untreated, will produce schizophrenia or Alzheimer's disease. From Dr. Randolph's view, food allergy and chemical susceptibilities are the root cause of many diseases. He correctly believed that one grain of any allergen—let's say one grain of wheat—will contaminate a huge batch of vitamins made from any other substance. It does not matter what the food is; the smallest amount imaginable is potent, if the patient is allergic to that specific food or to the chemicals sprayed upon the food. The particle that contaminated the new batch of vitamins will provoke physical and/or mental symptoms and other disease. Consequently, when I was his patient, Dr. Randolph did not recommend vitamins or minerals to any of his patients. Toward the end of his career he allowed cerebral-allergy patients to take very high-quality vitamin and mineral supplements. I cannot stress the importance of using the highest quality of vitamin and mineral supplementation that you can afford produced by laboratories that comply with the highest quality control standards obtainable. Purchase the most wholesome foods possible. Preferably, they will not have been sprayed with chemicals. If you have a garden, the

---

81 Every person in the world does better on his or her ancestral diet. See "Ancestral Diet" at http://www.hugnet.com.

ideal situation is to grow your own organic fruits and vegetables. Revitalize the garden with manure, compost and rock dust found near rock-crushing machinery in gravel pits. Rabbits and chickens provide meat and eggs. Let the chickens run around the garden. Their manure is an excellent source of fertilizer.

There is not the slightest doubt in my mind that if the patient has relatively few food allergies, he or she will be able to successfully do the four-day food rotation diet Dr. Randolph recommends. One of the troubles with this procedure is the initial expense of spending three weeks in an environmental allergy hospital unit. Most cerebral allergy patients lose their jobs and their insurance. Unless they are fortunate enough to participate in an adequate health insurance plan through a spouse's group coverage, or have independent means, the expense of going to a hospital allergy environmental unit is prohibitive. Twenty years ago, it cost our family approximately $14,000. In 2002 dollars, the $14,000 figure would be $45,000. In addition, the process of learning which foods provoke symptoms of disease is about as tough as going through army boot camp. It is certainly worth the money and effort, but it is not easy. Finally, if the allergy patient is allergic to too many foods, the four-day rotation diet is too difficult to follow. If a cerebral allergy patient must cook his or her meals, it is impossible. Over these last 20 years, better strategies to ameliorate the food allergy problem have been developed; so for most people, I do not recommend a strict rotation diet anymore.

Keep in mind that one of the first clinical signs most people tend to exhibit from low-level mercurial poisoning is allergy. At first a person might notice a minor problem with dust, pollens, flatulence and irritable bowel syndrome, or eruptions on the face and back of the neck that work their way down to both wrists. I remember asking one of my physicians at the onset of the Alzheimer's disease process, "Can a person be sick and not know it?" The internist did all kinds of tests for three weeks, but could find nothing wrong. Neither the physician nor patient recognizes the subject has been poisoned or connects mercury dental fillings to scores of different symptoms from wetting the bed to brain allergies, etc.[82] For three years, my health and short-term memory process continued to decline until I decided to get the Heidelberg Stomach Acid Test that indicated my stomach acid was more neutral than water. After the test, as I rounded the corner from the testing room to my physician's office, I saw Dr. David Buscher, Environmental Allergy, sitting at his desk looking at my tests results, shaking his head in stunned silence. That was the first breakthrough connecting short-term memory loss, brain-fog and brain-fag to allergy. Later I told Dr. Huggins that my stomach fluid pH was 7.2. He checked a group of his chronically ill dental patients for low stomach acid and found all of the mercury-toxic patients he tested had low stomach acid.

From my view, the easiest and most effective treatment protocol to eliminate food allergies is the treatment protocol that Dr. Sandra Denton uses. I think enough of her expertise that in December 1992 I drove the Alcan Highway from Anacortes, Washington, to Anchorage, Alaska,[83] to seek her services, and I have not needed to see an environmental allergist since that time. More importantly, Dr. Denton thoroughly understands the amalgam issue.

I never bothered to learn her treatment protocol, because the treatment process does not require patient participation. Dr. Denton resolved dozens, probably over 100 food allergies that made living a real chore. A friend, and one of my editors, Sandra Duffy, an attorney for the Multnomah County Attorneys Office in Portland, Oregon, thoroughly understands the treatment protocol and graciously offered to write the following information about this procedure for me. I quote her e-mail in its entirety, because I know this treatment process is the least expensive and easiest way to eliminate allergy symptoms.

"Re: Short exposition on the use of Nambudripad's Allergy Elimina-

---

82 When I became Dr. Randolph's patient at his environmental hospital in January of 1982, his patients had dozens of different symptoms of disease.

83 The clinic telephone number is (907) 563-6200.

tion Therapy (NAET) for mercury toxic/allergic symptoms.

"The ADA denies that mercury amalgam dental fillings cause any health harm other than an allergic reaction in very few hypersensitive people. While mercury is toxic to everybody, it actually does trigger an immune response in some.

"However, contrary to the ADA assertions, scientific studies show this immune reactivity is a very common phenomenon. One study revealed that 44% of fourth year dental students were immune reactive to dental amalgam. Clifford Testing data of thousands of patients showed that 93% were immune reactive to mercury amalgam.

"Many mercury-poisoned patients have found substantial symptom relief with an acupuncture-based treatment called Nambudripad's Allergy Elimination Therapy. Through Clifford testing, muscle testing, or other testing (never have a patch test for mercury) the practitioner can determine if a patient is immune reactive to mercury amalgams. If it is determined the patient is immune reactive to mercury amalgams, he holds a vial containing the offending allergen while the acupuncturist uses a mechanical stimulator on the spine, and then either inserts acupuncture needles at specific meridian points or manually stimulates those points. The patient then avoids the allergen to the best of his or her ability for at least 24 hours and occasionally rubs the acupuncture points. The patient can then be tested to see if the desensitization was successful. It generally is, but can be repeated if necessary.[84]

Sound kooky? It sure does. The bottom line is, it works! It works better than any allergy treatment I know, and I have tried them all. There isn't any allergy treatment protocol as effective as NAET.

---

84 For the names certified NAET practitiioners' contact: NAET, 6714 Beach Boulevard, Buena Park, CA 90621. (714) 523-8900, e-mail: naet@earthlink.net.

Candida Yeast Infection

Chronic low-level mercurial poisoning and sugar exacerbate yeast infection that causes leaky-gut syndrome.[85] The tissues of our intestines are approximately the size of a tennis court. Imagine a membrane that large, which under a microscope is so full of holes it looks like Swiss cheese. Several years ago a story circulated about a fellow in Japan who was arrested for driving while intoxicated who did not drink. His digestive system was so impaired, infected and run down that food fermentation manufactured alcohol in his intestine. If you have flatulence, if you tend to belch or require antacids for burning stomach sensations, the real culprit is not excessive acid. It is low, or, in many cases, no stomach acid. You need a Heidelberg stomach acid test for digestive enzymes and HCl. Food must digest properly to supply the brain with nutrients.

The food-allergy problem will never be satisfactorily resolved until the patient gets rid of all mercury fillings, fragments, mercury tattoos, root canals and jawbone infection, repairs the digestive process and really begins to chew his or her food. Otherwise chunks of food cannot digest properly, causing leaky-gut syndrome.

Why feed your enemy?

Think of it this way. If you were the U.S. President and your country had been a part of a coalition that went to war against an unprincipled psychopathic dictator who slaughtered his own citizens and invaded his neighbors, would you supply the maniac with the foodstuffs he needed to raise another healthy army to ferment further trouble? Then why would you feed candida? Candida craves sugar, starch, refined

---

85 The Merck Manual 17th Edition 1999, P 2636 "Mercury: Treatment: Observe for GI perforation."

flour and junk food. It will kill you if you allow it to. Your anti-tank shells are vegetable juice and raw green vegetables. M-16 rifle shells are cooked vegetables.

The fittest man I ever saw was Warren Moon, a Seahawk football player standing in the checkout line at a supermarket toward the end of his career. He had only one product in his sack, several pounds of kale. Warren was approximately 45 years old. He looked 25. Do you think Mr. Moon gets enough exercise? Then you, too, get off your duff and start walking. Pretend you are a lineman. Go for broke! Never, ever give up.

I won't deceive you: when you stop eating sugar and junk foods, expect to feel miserable for a few days. Do it anyway. Candida die-off raises Cain. It wants to live and you're killing it. Understand, sugar means refined flour and grains, especially rice, artificial sugar, sweet or starchy vegetables, sugared drinks and fruit juices. If you will not do this-and if anyone knows how difficult it is, it is I-there is little chance for recovery. Ninety-five percent of candida infection has to be eradicated before it is safe to eat sweets once in a while.

During World War II, food was in short supply in Japan and Allied prisoners-of-war diets were inadequate to maintain life. As the prisoners' health declined and their flesh wasted away, some of these men developed schizophrenia. Dr. Abram Hoffer, irrefutably the most knowledgeable orthomolecular psychiatrist in North America, treated the former soldiers with megadoses of vitamins. Schizophrenia remained in remission until they discontinued their vitamin regimen, particularly B3. They recovered when they resumed their course of treatment. This signifies that malnutrition is connected to mental disease.

Jawbone infection is also connected to schizophrenia and Alzheimer's disease. As is noted in Chapter 2, cavitations need to be identified and cleaned up for complete recovery from these diseases.

Surviving the Cure

Over the years I have studied the literature, searched the Internet and quietly listened to many others trying to discover a safe method to remove mercury from the brain. Your options are: (1) chelation, (2) homeopathic remedies and (3) hot baths.

What everybody needs to do is remove mercury from the body without causing further injury to themselves, or if that is not possible, to minimize the damage that does occur.

DMPS

Three chelation specialists I respect tell me DMPS (2, 3 dimercaptopropane sulfonate) is safe and has saved many lives. They also say DMPS should never be used in any patient who is deficient in trace minerals (determined by hair analysis), or the macro minerals, sodium, potassium, calcium and magnesium (readily evaluated by SMAC-23 or SMAC-24). Some mercury toxic patients told me DMPS worked very well for them. Others, including myself, have different stories. Insofar as I am able to determine, most brain allergy patients have low stomach acid and do not digest their food well, which causes a deficiency of the above trace and macro minerals. If the patient is suffering from brain fog, be sure to do the recommended tests. More than any other single factor in choosing to use, or not to use DMPS is the expertise of your physician.

Homeopathic Remedies

Dr. Huggins said that he found a cautionary reference about not using mercury to chelate mercury in an old homeopathic handbook. I have since learned that Dr. Huggins is correct. All dental amalgam should be removed from your teeth, gums and jawbone before taking the mercury homeopathic chelating agent or any other chelating program to remove mercury from the rest of your body. Homeopathic remedies to remove mercury from my body worked very well for me, but I had every mercury filling and amalgam fragment removed from my teeth, gums and jawbone before using the homeopathic remedy.

Saunas

Do not use public saunas. Every person in the sauna who has mercury fillings out-gasses mercury from their fillings. With every breath they take releases mercury into the air for others to absorb.

I do recommend either the hot water soak or the mud bath. Take your choice.

Hot Baths

Dr. Huggins recommends soaking in a hot bathtub at 104° for 20 minutes-just 20 minutes, not one degree higher or one minute longer than 20 minutes or you will heat the core temperature of your body too high. Cover yourself with a hot wet towel and place a wet hand towel over your head. Do this every day for six days. Rinse yourself off afterwards. I take a quick shower.

1. The first two days, add two cups of Epson salts to the bath water.

2. The third and fourth days, add one cup Epson salts and one cup baking soda.

3. The fifth and sixth days add two cups baking soda to the bath water and add one (1) pint of hydrogen peroxide to the bath water on the sixth day.

If you follow through faithfully, sooner or later the bath water or your bed sheets will suddenly turn gray. Repeat the program several months later. Keep in mind that I am not a medical professional. The only thing I can pass along is that I've tried just about everything I can think of to become mercury-free. What did I learn about chelation? Slow seems better than dumping mercury fast. Sending mercury directly to the skin is safer than allowing mercury to be reabsorbed by the liver.

Mud Baths

The mud I recommend is a special bentonite,[86] which is very likely the safest, quickest, easiest and least expensive way to chelate mercury, lead, aluminum, cadmium, arsenic and carbon monoxide from the body. I wish this product had been available 17 years ago. Carefully read all of the literature about it. Keep in mind that I am only speaking for myself. You need to make your own decisions about your treatment process.

How To Get Well Again

If I were you, and you are as sick as I was at the beginning of my illness, I would do whatever it takes to get well. These are 28 steps that worked for me. Material Biocompatibility Blood tests were in process of being developed by Dr. Huggins and I was too ill to put off treatment one day longer. I had all my teeth extracted by an oral surgeon. For everyone else, these are the 28 steps that worked for me.

1. Replace Fillings or Pull Teeth

What's more important: your brain or your teeth? The average American dental patient has 12 amalgam dental fillings. Huge amounts of mercury are released while old fillings are being drilled out. Dead

86 See Appendix IV.

brain tissue is found in spinal fluid for 24 hours after a mercury amalgam filling has been replaced. If the patient has a lot of mercury-amalgam dental work in the mouth or is gravely ill, I think the safest, best and least expensive solution would be to have a really good oral surgeon pull all of their teeth and meticulously clean the resulting cavitations. Every mercury filling, tattoo and fragment of amalgam in your mouth, gums or jawbone as well as infection within the jawbone must be removed before your immune system can regain enough strength to begin the healing process. Only highly trained professionals realize the importance of these procedures.

"If I were diagnosed with an incurable degenerative disease, I would definitely extract any questionable teeth. I would never leave a root canal in a person considered terminal. The infected tooth you leave could be the one that is killing the patient."

— Dr. Harold Ravin

"Dr. Weston Price's work shows how germs become trapped in dentin tubules and accessory root canals. While dentists sterilize the root canal, there are over three miles of inaccessible, untreated tubules from which germs can pour toxins into your body. These poisons can affect your heart, kidneys, lungs, eyes, stomach, brain, and countless other body tissues. At times, the germs themselves escape into the bloodstream and are carried throughout the body."

— Dr. Jerry Mittelman

2. Finding the Right Dentist

Finding a really good mercury-free dentist is more important to the recovery process than any other single thing that I could do. I had 26 mercury dental fillings, several gold crowns and a bridge. I have never been sorry that I had all my teeth extracted. That is what I would do again. The action you choose should depend on the amount of dental work in your mouth.

3. Biocompatibility Tests

I would definitely get a biocompatibility blood test because the only thing that belongs in our mouths is our own teeth. There are no dental materials that are biocompatible for everyone. Some mercury-toxic dental patients are allergic to all metals. Many of the old men I see, fellows in their late 80s and early 90s who still play golf, have high-quality gold fillings in their mouths. All of them are healthy and none of them appear to have diminished thought process. One caution: If necessary, use compatible temporary fillings, but get all of the mercury out of your teeth, gums and jawbone before using gold. Gold absorbs mercury like a sponge.

4. What's More Expensive?

Initially, gold is more expensive than mercury or composite fillings. Over the rest of your life, insofar as mercury-free dentists can determine, and provided these metals pass your individual biocompatibility blood test,[87] 82 percent 24-karat gold combined with 18 percent platinum is the best, least expensive dental filling material available. People think nothing of buying new high-end automobiles. What is your health worth? Before it's over, mercury poisoning will probably cost four generations of our family, the state of Washington and the Federal Government a minimum of 7 million dollars in unnecessary hospital, welfare, social service and medical expenses. It will be the end of our bloodline. None of my children have children. Why would any sane person risk passing schizophrenia or Alzheimer's disease to their progeny? From a personal view, mercury poisoning from dental fillings

---

87 Do not run right out and use gold, or any other dental material, until they have been screened and you do not react to these materials. All mercury fillings must be removed from your mouth before you allow the dentist to use gold. In addition, 3% of the population is allergic to gold and 1% is allergic to platinum. Some dental patients are allergic to all metals.

cost me a lifetime of missed opportunity. That's the real price of mercury amalgam dental fillings and root canals. By comparison, the cost of high-quality gold is insignificant.

5. False Teeth

If I decided to have false teeth, I would not allow the dentures to be colored. The pink color in dentures is mercuric sulfide. I'd exchange a root canal for a bridge. I would require the resin be dried at low temperature for at least 11 hours to allow the monomer and polymer to be released from the resin. Dental lab technicians tend to cut drying time, which will cause your mouth to blister and burn due to allergic reaction to monomers and polymers. Those substances are also released if dental plates are dried in a vacuum. My dentist made a mold of my teeth. Not even my twin sister realized that I had false teeth until I told her. Save the mold. If you chip or break a false tooth, you may need it later.

6. After an Extraction

If I accidentally lost a blood clot in a tooth socket, I would immediately return to the dental office to reclean the infection and cause bleeding. New bone is formed from blood. Remember, all dry sockets will become reinfected. Waste products from anaerobic bacteria living in jawbone and root canal infection are poisonous.

7. Dental Appointments

Consecutive seven-day dental appointments seriously stress the immune system. Receptionists like to schedule dental appointments at the same time on the same day each week because it is easier for the patient to remember to keep an appointment. Staggering appointments is better, however. The immune system seems to work on a 21 seven-day cycle (day 7, day 14, day 21). The trauma of dental treatment suppresses the immune system on the first appointment. A second seven-day appointment can suppress the immune system further. On the 21st day, the immune system needs to rest and refresh itself or the patient's immune system can be destabilized. If you make a dental appointment on Monday, schedule the second weekly appointment no earlier than Wednesday and the third appointment on Tuesday or Friday.

8. Support

I would join Dental Amalgam Mercury Syndrome, Inc. (DAMS), a national group. You will find support and practical advice from people with similar problems. Their telephone numbers and addresses will be found in Appendix IX.

9. Digestive Enzymes And HCl.

I have taken digestive enzymes and HCl (hydrochloric acid) for more than 15 years.

10. To Cure Depression

Releasing mercury quickly during the drilling process may cause the dental patient to slip into deep depression without recognizing the signs. Walking up and down hills for three days cases depression to evaporate. After a tooth is extracted, allow three days for the blood clots to stay put, then start your exercise again.[88]

88 Do not tense the muscles in your face. Do not jog for two weeks. Give blood clots time to heal.

11. Walking to Wellness

So far dentists, environmental physicians and your support team have done most of the work to help you recover. This is the part that decides who lives and who dies. There is no use asking anyone else for help. You're on your own. If you sit back and expect others to bail you out, right up front, you're headed for a psychiatric hospital or had better get your affairs in order. So no matter how unwell you feel at the moment, pull up your socks, tighten your belt, start walking and get on with getting well. Never, ever give up!

In 18 months, you will wonder why you thought paying the price to recover was so difficult.

12. Overcoming Fatigue

Fatigue makes cowards of us all. If necessary, sit on a trampoline and bounce each day until you regain enough energy to stand. For months, I had to crawl up a flight of stairs and rest twice to reach the second floor. The most difficult thing to do was the struggle to push one foot ahead of the other. It took a half-hour to walk 50 yards. The back of my shirt would be soaked in sweat. Unless you literally cannot stand up, walk. If you can only walk 100 feet, start putting one foot ahead of the other. Go! Tomorrow walk 110 feet. Keep right on going. Do not worry about brain-fog, how bad you feel or how difficult it is: walk! If you walk far enough, your thought process will clear, depression will cease and you will become an easier-going, more considerate person.

Eventually we moved near the sea and I walked up and down hills in a beautiful park three and a half to seven miles at least three times, sometimes four times a week. Wherever you walk, avoid automobile exhaust. For several months before we moved. I walked up and down hills after midnight to avoid the traffic. Vehicle exhaust fumes contain trace amounts of mercury and cyanide.

Along these same lines, a really good internist's wife had a disease he was unable to diagnose. The only thing the physician knew was that she was dying. He made her walk. At first she could walk less than 100 feet. Now, they close their office for lunch and walk. In the evening after dinner, they walk another hour. When I met the physician's wife again, she was radiantly healthy.

13. A Lifesaving Rule

Remember the following rule; if you smell any obnoxious odor, immediately remove the offending substance away from you, or you away from it. Your nose knows. It is your first line of defense. Pay attention to what it is telling you. You are low on trace minerals and it will take months of taking a little swig of trace minerals every day before you will notice any improvement. In a year, provided you have taken trace minerals every day, odors will cease being troublesome.

14. Water

I would purchase a high-quality whole-house water filter to remove chlorine and contaminants from drinking water, sinks, bathtubs and showers, toilets and the washing machine. Exposures to chlorine, underarm deodorant and hair spray caused me to become an explosive jackass. I caused so much needless turmoil and pain to our family.

If it was just chlorine, getting well would be easy, but all sorts of chemicals and foods, particularly favorite foods, are problematic. Installing a whole-house water filter is expensive. It is a real challenge to come up with the money to build an uncontaminated living environment.

15. Avoid Nutrition Zappers.

Stop consuming sugar, artificial sweeteners,[89] junk food, coffee and soda pop. Expect to feel miserable for a few days. Grit your teeth. Pull up your socks and WALK to sweat the poisons out! Drink at least two quarts of water every day. If you do not have a water filter, boil water on the stove to allow chlorine to evaporate.

16. Eat Organic, Avoid Chemicals

Insofar as possible, I would try not to eat chemicalized foodstuffs. If possible, eat organic foods instead.

17. Avoid Fish

Stop eating fish, especially large bottom fish, tuna and shellfish. If one has mercury poisoning, most of the fish in our oceans, lakes and rivers are too polluted with mercury and chemical contamination to eat fish anymore.

18. Nutritional Supplements

I would immediately begin to take vitamins, minerals, and trace minerals, and I would take digestive enzymes every time I put food in my mouth, every single day for the rest of my life. The food supplements I take will be found in Appendix II.

---

89 As substitute sweeteners metabolize, during the next to the last process they turn into formaldehyde. Then they turn into alcohol. Using substitute sugar is a case of jumping from the frying pan into the fire.

19. Stop Eating Junk Food

Learn which foods provoke brain-fog and brain-fag and begin to rotate foods. This is the most difficult part of the healing process. Unless the reader does this one thing-and it takes real work-it is unlikely they will be able to recover. In the beginning of my illness, Alzheimer's disease, I was allergic to 141 from a list of 145 foods. No food allergy test that I took indicated that I had more than four free-foods (foods that did not provoke brain-fog or brain-fag). Carefully read about food allergy. It is a key to unlocking a clear thought process and reversing dozens of dissimilar diseases. Keep in mind that food allergies and chemical sensitivities are not the cause of your distress. They are a symptom of an overloaded weakened immune system. Heavy metal poisoning, root canals, cavitations, chemical toxicity and, in some cases, mold are the underlying cause of your distress.

20. A Useful Book

I would purchase my first book, *Beating Alzheimer's*. This book, *Reversing Chronic Disease* covers a huge area of medicine. Chapter 3 is primarily aimed at the Alzheimer's sufferer who needs the least complicated information possible to recover. *Beating Alzheimer's* covers food allergy and chemicals in more detail.

21. Sleep

This may seem a little silly, but get a good night's sleep. Sleep deprivation causes depression and muddled thinking. Sleeping during regular nighttime hours in a dark room promotes melatonin production that helps protect against mercury toxicity. Deep, healthy sleep promotes healing of the immune system.

22. Clothing

The preferable clothing of choice is 100 percent cotton, wool or silk. Synthetic materials provoke brain-fog. One of the best pieces of clothing that chemically sensitive patients can wear to lounge around the house in is100 percent cotton sweats. They are inexpensive and easy to care for. Assuming you wear cotton underwear, slip the elastic band of your shorts over the cotton T-shirt. Otherwise you will become allergic to elastic.

23. The Home Environment

We love our view of the mountains. We have a well-built, lovely condominium. I took a chance purchasing it. Because of my age, the fact that I had middle-age onset diabetes, two minor heart attacks (AF), two strokes, and have kidney disease, I do not anticipate a prolonged existence. Louise does not have chemical sensitivity. Her mercury fillings were replaced years ago. I think she will do well here. Nonetheless, if I notice out-gassing fumes from the furnace, or develop dark shiners under my eyes near the nose that indicate petroleum fumes are becoming a problem, we will move. I should have exchanged the gas furnace and our gas hot water heater for an electric furnace immediately. It is too late to do that now. Petrochemical fumes have contaminated the air vents. If there had been a gas stove in the kitchen or a gas water heater in the living area, we would not have purchased the condominium under any circumstances. I cover this subject in more detail in *Beating Alzheimer's*. If this was an older home that had an old gas furnace, if the dwelling did not have an air exchanger, or if it were located near a busy street, we wouldn't have considered buying it. Move at least three miles from a freeway. Be careful which way the prevailing winds blow. If the wind blows across a freeway or from an industrial area toward the prospective dwelling you are considering, walk away from the deal. It's not for you.

24. Toxins From Publications

I would move newspapers, books, magazines and other printed material out of the living areas of the home, particularly from the bedrooms. I would stop subscribing to newspapers and watch the early news on television. But I would not watch television more than one or two hours per day. Don't become a fat depressed couch potato.

25. Cleaning Products

With the exception of one can of Bon Ami® scouring powder, a sponge and an unscented dishwashing detergent and one bar of mild hand soap, I would remove all other chemicals from under the sinks.

26. Petrochemical Fumes

I would park the automobile outside of the home. Never park an automobile under a bedroom. Petroleum fumes rise. If the garage connects to the house, take all of the chemicals out of the garage to an outside storage shed or, better yet, throw them away and do not buy them anymore.

27. Carpets

I would never purchase multicolored synthetic carpets. Every time the carpet manufacturer adds a color, the carpet is dipped into formaldehyde again.

28. Indoor Plants

Place several spider plants, peace lilies or Chinese evergreens in the home to reduce toxic chemical contamination.

That's it: This is what I would do. It is not easy. It takes a while, but if you stick with the program you should be able to regain your health. Do not forget to thank the Lord that He put this information in your hands.

Chapter 4

Recovery Stories

These are the histories of people who have recovered from supposedly irreversible chronic diseases after removal of their mercury dental fillings and root canals. I could have included many other similar stories, but it isn't necessary. The cat is out of the bag and the ADA can't put it back.

1. Louise's Story

As the articles about Alzheimer's state, the disease is insidious and hard to recognize at first. The symptoms are vague and you wonder if there is really something wrong, and/or what is wrong? All too soon you are certain something is not right and you pray that it's not what you have begun to suspect.

My husband, Tom, was having memory problems and began to react in anger to the slightest provocation. As his memory declined, I was becoming more frustrated. He would repeatedly ask the same question. After the third time within a few minutes, I would ask Tom: "Don't you remember you just asked me that?" It was at this point I insisted Tom see a doctor who sent him for a CAT (Computer axial topography) scan.

On June 13, 1983, which was also the day that our daughter graduated from high school, we heard the diagnosis-Alzheimer's disease.

Our initial response was utter hopelessness.

The following week there was a "20/20" Barbara Walters special on television about Alzheimer's disease we were anxious to see. The program left us more depressed than ever, especially since Tom remembered Rita Hayworth, who also had Alzheimer's disease, as a beautiful, talented actress. Understanding how little was known about the disease and that medicine had no idea how to help the patient was devastating.

Then Tom took a tour of the Alzheimer's ward at Western State Hospital at Fort Steilacoom, Washington. Whether this was a wise move is debatable. Fortunately, Tom's value system forbids suicide. His first thought was that he would rather die any other way.

A period of deep depression followed. Tom hoped to die quickly. When this did not happen after a period of time, he prayed that through him the cure for Alzheimer's be found.

At the time, Tom was 50 years old.[90] I was 39. Tom's mother had spells of mental illness and obvious memory problems. (When Tom's AD first occurred, we did not connect his mother being a dental assistant to her ailments.) She died at 92. The physician told Tom that he might have as long as seven years to live. The prospect was not something that I could dwell on. I refused to think about the probable outcome. We made a decision not to sit back and wait for the inevitable. The future was too bleak to accept.

Being a pharmacist, I understood the published research papers. Reading every pharmacy article relating to AD didn't give any encouragement. Almost all of the writing was directed to managing the patient or how to cope with the stress of being a caregiver. Ironically, books on AD still have this same theme.

We frequented health food stores buying books about problems simi-

---

90 October 8th 2003, Tom was 71 years old.

lar to Tom's symptoms. Tom could understand what he read and would mark anything that seemed important because he couldn't remember the ideas more than a few seconds. I reviewed the same material in the evening after I returned from work. By this time Tom had not been able to work for a while. He frequently had to look up our own telephone number and I quickly learned to be careful where I parked because it was very difficult for him to find our automobile in parking lots.

If anything suggested possibilities, we investigated carefully. Tom went to physicians who were referred to as being pre-eminent within their specialties in the books that we read. Some things seemed to help. Others were a waste of time and money.

This has been a lengthy learning experience. Our search started with allergies including inhalants and foods. Tom tried acupuncture, different nutrition ideas and a half-dozen other things. A homeopathic physician helped in the beginning. Then, in May of 1985, Tom asked Dr. David Buscher to give him a Heidelberg stomach acid test that indicated he had no stomach acid. He began taking betaine HCl and digestive enzymes along with certain vitamins and minerals. In 1986 we learned there is mercury in silver amalgam dental fillings through an article in the Seattle Well Mind Association newsletter.[91] Tom tried replacing all of the silver fillings in his mouth, but that was before Dr. Huggins' dental materials biocompatible blood test was available and composite fillings caused severe swelling for weeks. At that point Tom had an oral surgeon remove all of his teeth and amalgam fragments within his gums and jawbone.

In June of 1987, four years after the original diagnosis of Alzheimer's disease, a second CAT scan revealed the markers pinpointing Alzheimer's disease were absent.[93] Later we learned about cavita-

---

91 Well Mind Association, 4649 Sunnyside Avenue North, #344, Seattle, Washington, 98103.

92 There is slight residual damage to the brain due to an automobile accident at age five.

tions, jawbone infections, and Tom had over 20 infected sites cleaned up, which further improved his memory and disposition. The journey is basically over, but we continue to read and learn and to take nutritional supplements.

The stress of living with and caring for someone with Alzheimer's has been both emotional and financial. Unfortunately, I discovered that I am a stress eater and I gained 80 pounds during this time. Tom was not easy to live with. About one-third of people who have Alzheimer's become argumentative, antagonistic and develop dementia. This type of irrational behavior is predictable pathology of the Alzheimer's disease process. Tom's personality change decimated our entire family. As his wife, I made a commitment in sickness and in health. And, I remembered how my husband used to be. In June 2002, we were able to celebrate our 38th anniversary. It was a lovely day, Tom is easier-going again, almost like his old self, and I'm thankful that we both are aware of each other and enjoy living again.

Tom is reasonably well, but his immune system has been damaged, so he has to be somewhat careful of his lifestyle. He changed careers and has become a writer with zeal to help others. A large research grant for AD was funded, in part, because of his book being published in 1989.

It is especially rewarding to hear from other people who have recovered after reading *Beating Alzheimer's*. These letters make my day. One thank-you note left me in tears. It reminded me how fortunate we are. I thank God that he has seen us through this struggle.

Here is a chronology of Tom's doctor and dental visits put together from old insurance records. They are not all-inclusive, because most of the physicians he went to are not considered mainstream medical doctors whose treatments were not covered by insurance and there is no record of many office calls. Neither does one time period necessarily mean one office visit. It means Tom went to that particular doctor during the time periods listed below. Every physician referred to is an expert in his or her own field of practice.

1981 Dr. Richard Wilkerson, Environmental Medicine, Yakima, WA.

1981 Dr. David Buscher, Environmental Medicine, Bellevue, WA.

1981 Dr. Eloise Kailen (deceased), Environmental Medicine, Sequim, WA.

1982 Dr. Theron Randolph (deceased), Environmental Allergy Hospital Unit, Henrotin Hospital, Chicago, IL (23 days).

1983 Dr. Richard Wilkerson, Environmental Medicine, Yakima, WA.

1983 Diagnosis of Alzheimer's disease, St. Peter Hospital. Olym pia, WA.

1984 Dr. Dean Crothers, Homeopathy, Edmonds, WA.

1985 Dr. David Buscher, Environmental Medicine, Bellevue, WA.

1986 Dr. Eloise Kailen (above)

1986 Dr. Hal Huggins, testing for mercury toxicity, at that time in Colorado Springs, CO.

1986 Dr. Ron Pinson, Conventional Oral Surgeon, Anacortes, WA.

1988 Dr. Hal Huggins,[93] to remove 20 jawbone infections (cavitations).

1991 Dr. Russell Jaffe, Princeton Bio Center, Blood tests for nutritional deficiencies, Skillman, NJ.

1991 Dr. Sandra Denton, Environmental Medicine, Mercury Toxicity Specialist, Nutritional Medicine and allergy specialist, Anchorage, Alaska (20 days). Tom has not needed to see any environmental allergy physician since becoming Dr. Denton's patient ten years ago.

---

93 http://www.hugnet.com/

1998 Dr. Jonathan Collin, [94] Nutritional Medicine and Chelation Specialist, Editor of the Townsend Letter for Doctors and Patients.

Tom saw many other physicians and alternative-practice specialists. Over the last 20-plus years we have moved seven times and we are unable to remember many office calls and doctor's names. If you are new in town, one of the best places to find a really competent physician is to ask a pharmacist. If you are seeking an alternative practitioner, ask health food storeowners for references. Customers tend to brag about competent health care providers. If you have chronic disease, find an alternative-practice physician and dentist. One of the best medical practitioners Tom knows is Dr. Horst Poehlmann, who told him, "Doctors hate me. My patients love me." If we lived in Australia, that's the doctor Tom would go to.

---

2. Elaine Umstead's Story

We both went to the Huggins Diagnostic Center in Colorado Springs, Colorado, August 21, 1990, for the most beneficial investment of time and money we have ever spent. Al was getting the mercury from his dentures. The pink coloring in dental plates has been identified as mercury.

His new dentures are now set in clear acrylic and the change in Al is incredible. Dr. Huggins had never seen such a change in any other patient in just one week. As we follow Dr. Huggins' program, the improvement continues. I had arranged to put Al in a board-and-care home because I could no longer deal with him. I am most delighted to say I called and canceled the reservation. Al began a second series of chelation September 7, 1990, and the improvement continues.

I am so grateful for your book, conversations, and suggestions. You

---

94 http://www.drjonathancollin.com/

have literally saved Al's life. Thank you! It is incredible how things we have about us we do not really think about affect us.

---

3. Cardiovascular and Peripheral Vascular Disease

Dr. F. Fuller Royal reports in the May 1990 Townsend Letter for Doctors and Patients that one of his patients, H.R., suffered debilitating cardiovascular and peripheral vascular disease and was on oxygen almost continually. The patient was unable to walk across the room without experiencing severe angina pain in his chest.

Double bypass surgery had been performed in 1972, a second in 1978. The gentleman had three hospitalizations in 1984 for angina and a third bypass surgery was recommended. H.R. was not improving even though he was taking 10 drugs prescribed by his doctors. Believing there had to be a better way, his family rejected the advice of the specialists and took the patient to a Nevada clinic for evaluation and treatment. More than anything else, what H.R. really needed was a competent dentist. When 4 volts of direct current (DC) was externally applied at acupuncture points, the impedance was easily identified at tooth 17, a wisdom tooth in the left lower jaw interfering with the biochemical activity of heart tissue that continually stressed the heart muscle. After tooth 17 was extracted and the patient's prescription drugs were greatly reduced, within six months H.R. was able to walk four and one half miles a day.

---

4. Short-Term Memory Loss and Root Canals

A physician who had retired due to short-term memory loss had 13 root canals. He read the first edition of *Beating Alzheimer's* and pestered me time and again for further evidence that, if he was to have any chance for recovery, he needed to have all of his teeth removed. It isn't possible to bridge 13 root canals. For six months he checked and rechecked with mercury-free dentists and physicians from all over the world mentioned in *Beating Alzheimer's* before he went ahead. After his teeth were pulled, he went home and lay down on his bed expecting to die. He said, "I awoke two hours later. It was the first time in years my head was clear."

---

5. Leukemia

The first editor of *Beating Alzheimer's*, a family relative who had leukemia, was expected to die within three months. He did not believe a word of the information in my manuscript. Luckily, his teeth fell out and he lived another ten years. Dr. Huggins was speaking at a dental convention and mentioned silver amalgam's (mercurial poisoning's) connection to cancer. A physician in the audience turned white at the news because several years before, he was dying of leukemia and became so ill his teeth, which contained many mercury fillings, fell out. His cancer went into remission.

---

6. Tongue Cancer

A dentist prevented a dental hygienist from telling her patient she suspected the cause of the cancer on his tongue, right next to an enormous silver filling, was mercury toxicity. She quit.

---

7. Addy's Story

Several years ago, Addy told me her story after a speaking engagement. She had lost most of her short-term memory. She had hip pain, depression and chronic fatigue. Luckily she was still able to read *Beating Alzheimer's* and sought out a mercury-free dentist. Back pain ceased when the first root canal was extracted. She replaced all of her mercury-silver amalgam fillings, recovered from depression and regained her short-term memory. She is full of energy. I saw Addy about

18 months ago. She is healthier than I am. She is probably more well than her doctor. I smile and chuckle to myself every time I think of her, because I'm a little jealous.

---

8. This former patient prefers not to use her name

A young woman was dying by the hour. Area surgeons refused to operate. Dr. Denton located a corporate jet to fly her patient from Seattle, Washington, to Colorado Springs, Colorado. Two oral surgeons removed titanium implants within the lower jaw and all of her silver fillings. Both oral surgeons laughed at Dr. Denton. They told her the patient would die on the operating table, but she began to recover two hours after surgery. Six months later, this vain young woman had two titanium posts reimplanted into her jaw to anchor her lower dentures in place. She rapidly became schizophrenic. Dr. Denton pleaded with her surgeons to remove the implants, which they did, and she quickly recovered. Several years have gone by and the woman leads a normal life.

---

9. The Horse's Mouth-MS Recovery

I overheard two mainstream ADA dentists talking about an MS patient who recovered in one of their offices within minutes after one of them removed her mercury fillings. They were flabbergasted. I could have told them similar stories about other MS patients who had the same experience. Some MS patients, who were so ill I do not understand how they could have stayed alive, recovered after their mercury fillings were replaced with biocompatible materials. The ADA and Multiple Sclerosis Society both know this statement is true. They have seen Dr. Huggins' videotapes. Dr. Huggins had MS himself. Our family dentist told me about one of his MS patients who could barely crawl into the dental chair who, after removal of his mercury fillings, walked over and paid his bill before leaving the office. MS patients should not expect similar results from their former family dentist. You have special requirements, which ought to be used during amalgam removal, and every single ADA dentist who follows the party line needs to be retrained. You're not playing tiddlywinks; maybe no one can help, but the bet on the table is how you will live out the rest of your life. Get an expert.

So many others . . .

Over the last decade many people suffering short-term memory loss have told me that I saved their life. I never tried to keep count of the number of Alzheimer's patients who recovered and I will not suggest an exact figure because I don't know the answer. If I were pushed for an estimate, the figure would certainly be more than 50, probably less than 100. People cannot get in touch with me anymore because I became a recluse 11 years ago. So many Alzheimer's sufferers and worried relatives cost us so much energy, time and money that it was impossible to live a normal family life. All we could do was move and change our unlisted telephone number five or six times before life began to return to normal.

Personal medical histories from the Internet as told by their authors.[95]

---

10. 15 years of pain and suffering

Between the ages of four and six, I had six mercury amalgams placed in my mouth to fill cavities in my baby teeth. Just after placement of the first amalgams, I developed severe allergies to milk, terrible gas pains in my chest, persistent upper respiratory infections, and chronic

---

95 I do not personally know any of these people. These are their stories.

eczema, where the skin cracked and bled. These troubles continued until the age of 16, when I began to experience severe constipation and amenhorrea. At 18, I developed bleeding hemorrhoids, and by 20, I had acid reflux, and occasions of projectile vomiting.

At 23, I experienced two bouts of optic neuritis, and subsequent testing confirmed a diagnosis of multiple sclerosis. At 25, I began to have seizures—a burning, freezing sensation spread down my left side to my waist, my legs grew numb, and I became paralyzed from the waist down. The seizures, lasting one to two minutes, occurred anywhere from 5 to 15 times a day, and within eight months had disappeared. For the next five years I had the constant sensation my rectum was falling through my pelvic floor, and my problems with constipation and hemorrhoids worsened.

At 30, I started having incontinence and terrible muscle spasms throughout my lower back and pelvic floor, which pinched surrounding nerves, causing terrible pain. My digestive problems worsened, and I began to lose weight. My gastroenterologist diagnosed me with irritable bowel syndrome. Finally, at 31, in constant pain and with swollen abdomen, I started to have severe diarrhea, fever, and rectal bleeding. I was given a fissurectomy, but my condition worsened. Hospitalized, tests revealed I had bleeding ulcers throughout my lower intestines, fistulas forming abscesses in my abdominal cavity, and severe anemia. My supposed fissure was actually a bleeding rectal ulcer. I was diagnosed with Crohn's disease, and treated with steroids and antibiotics. Standing 5'5" tall, in just one year, my weight had dropped from 125 to 95 pounds.

In November of 1997, a month after starting treatment for Crohn's, I developed shingles, from activation of the Herpes Zoster virus. After the sores cleared, I suffered the burning, searing nerve pain of post-herpetic neuralgia for another two years. Four months into Crohn's treatment, I had a complete rectal prolapse — eight inches of my lower intestines fell from my anus and dangled inside out between my legs. Doctors surgically removed 12 inches of diseased colon and explored my abdominal cavity for cancer, but found nothing. While in the hospital, I suffered a grand mal seizure, which doctors were unable to explain.

After surgery, my health continued to deteriorate. My pain intensified, as constant muscle spasms pinched nerves, and neuralgia wracked my body. I had pains in my chest, back, and abdomen, and I became jaundiced. I suffered from chronic insomnia, short-term memory loss, and again, severe constipation. I developed terrible food allergies to dairy, wheat, gluten, corn, soy, eggs, preservatives, spices, sugar, and caffeine, which made the pain I felt after eating, and during digestion, excruciating. I lost even more weight. I also became allergic to all 17 of my medications, and was forced to stop taking them.

Desperate, I turned to alternative therapies, and found an acupuncturist and Doctor of Oriental Medicine in Los Angeles, who has developed a sensitive diagnostic technique to detect hidden pathogens causing illness. I began flying back and forth to Los Angeles from San Francisco for treatment and, for the first time in five years, began to improve. In October of 1998, after two months on Chinese herbs, I felt better overall, but I started to experience numbness in my legs and difficulty walking.

A week after the numbness started, I began having violent seizures involving my entire body. I lost all muscle control and thrashed wildly about the floor. My jaws ground back and forth, and I yawned repeatedly. During the third seizure, my jaw dislocated and I was rushed to the emergency room to have it reset. After two days, the seizures were constant and I was hospitalized in an attempt to control them; none of the medications worked. The neurologists had never seen anything like it and could offer no remedy. After three days under heavy sedation, my insurance company denied me further benefits, and I was discharged into the care of a psychiatrist, who tried an experimental antipsychotic drug not approved by the FDA. The drug's side effects exacerbated my existing symptoms.

I begged that my family return me to the OMD in Los Angeles, and I moved into a hotel near his office where, no longer in any condition to travel or take care of myself, I lived for eight months, the first three under the constant care of a family member. Soon after the move, I became paralyzed from the neck down, retaining only partial use of my right arm. I lost control of my facial features, tongue and mouth so that speech was nearly impossible. Sometimes, I was unable to open my eyes or to speak and could move only the pinky on my right hand to indicate I had not lost consciousness. Day and night, I kept a piece of wood between my teeth to prevent my jaw from dislocating again. The pain from the post-herpetic neuralgia was exquisite. I felt as if my skin had been burned away, and as if I was being probed with an electric cattle prod.

After clearing multiple layers of bacterial, viral and fungal infections, high levels of mercury were detected in my brain, spinal cord, and intestinal tract, causing autoimmune reactions. The source of mercury poisoning had come primarily from the dental amalgams placed in my baby teeth, 32 years before. Although my last filling had fallen out by the age of eight, the mercury remained, having entered my system through my lungs, sinuses, and intestinal tract, eventually permeating my entire body. The MS and Crohn's disease were caused by my immune system attempting to eliminate both the mercury and the multiple bacterial, viral, and fungal infections.

Blood tests and hair analysis by a Western physician specializing in heavy metal poisoning confirmed I had not only accumulated high levels of mercury from my teeth fillings, but also nickel, another heavy metal used in dental work. Because his treatment for clearing mercury, DMSA, increased the risk of seizure, he advised me to continue using Chinese herbs. As I began to clear mercury, I developed even more symptoms. Mercury re-activated the Herpes Zoster virus, causing my optic neuritis to flare again, and I developed painful hearing sensitivities and ringing in my ears. I became extremely sensitive to odors of any kind, the slightest smell making it difficult for me to breathe, and provoking a seizure. At other times, in episodes lasting between ten and twenty seconds, my diaphragm froze. I could neither inhale nor exhale, although I consciously directed myself to.

Mercury in my lungs was blocking the nerve impulse transmissions between my brain and diaphragm. Two weeks after a modification to my herbal prescription, the difficulties with my diaphragm disappeared, and gradually, as I cleared more mercury, my problems with vision, hearing and smell were also resolved.

After two months of taking herbal prescriptions to clear mercury, the paralysis began to recede from my upper torso and I could use my arms to lift myself up out of my wheelchair. I regained some feeling in my legs and could drag myself across a room, or help myself in and out of bed. The constant movements I was having in my limbs, and loss of control of my tongue and facial muscles, were symptoms of Tardive Dyskinesia, a condition of the central nervous system found in individuals having taken high dosages of antipyschotic drugs over long periods of time. These drugs chelate manganese; however, in my case, mercury had interfered with the function of both molybdenum and magnesium in my brain, producing the same dysfunction. Magnesium regulates neuromuscular contractions and has important anti-seizure effects on the body. I began taking supplements of both, while continuing with herbs to clear mercury, and soon the symptoms of Tardive Dyskinesia disappeared completely, my nerve pain improved, and my seizures became less violent.

The seizures also changed character. Instead of grand sweeping movements, I became either rigid, or twitched incessantly, as my body shook with tremors. I had petit mal seizures, where, with frozen stare, I sat in a trance-like state. My joints swelled and became stiff, throbbing with arthritic pain, and my hands and feet curled up into claws. The painful muscle spasms in my back, legs, and pelvic floor returned. Mercury was found blocking both calcium channels and hormone receptors, and mercury antibodies had triggered an autoimmune attack on joint tissue.

Finally, after four months of clearing mercury, the neurological issues began to abate. The paralysis in my hips and legs slowly receded, and after five months I could walk with a cane, and soon after with no assistance at all. My seizures and tremors stopped, the numbness and nerve pain diminished, and my joint pain relented. By May of 1999, the neurological issues had cleared, but instead, I began another exacerbation of Crohn's disease. The debilitating diarrhea with fever returned, as I had 40 to 50 attacks a day, and abdominal cramping left me doubled over in pain. Mercury-related microfistulas were found along my entire digestive tract, from my esophagus to my rectum, once again causing pockets of infection in my abdominal cavity.

Though still terribly weak, I moved home to San Francisco in late June of 1999, and again traveled to Los Angeles to continue treatment. Gradually, as I improved, my food allergies abated and my weight came up to 99 pounds. Because the fistulas were slow to heal, in September and October of 1999, under the supervision of my gastroenterologist, I underwent three infusions of Remicaide, a new Crohn's medication that specifically targets treatment-resistant fistulas. The results were positive.

Today, after 20 months of clearing mercury, my intestinal issues are mild, my neurological difficulties are non-existent, my food allergies gone (although I continue to avoid all dairy), and, at 115 pounds, my weight has returned to normal. I take a yoga class every other day, and 30-minute walks three times a week. At 34, I am feeling better than I have in 15 years. Although I am still clearing residues of mercury, and continue my trips to Los Angeles for treatment, I anticipate once I am completely free of mercury and its related antibodies, I will enjoy a full and permanent recovery.

---

11. One Silver Amalgam Filling

My own brush with mercury intoxication from just one dental filling may not be the most dramatic case that you will read, but it has almost the simplicity of a lab experiment. One amalgam filling (my first ever, at age 40) was put in, symptoms appeared almost immediately, the filling was replaced with a composite (non-mercury) filling four months later, and the symptoms disappeared.

I have enjoyed excellent health all my life. I'm a Minnesota boy and I always prided myself on being able to take the nastiest, coldest or rainiest weather. Tough and athletic, I ran the mile in high school and have always been energetic. But in January 1985, my health suddenly changed. What follows is based on my notes from a diary that I kept.

On January 9, 1985, a dentist put the first silver filling in my mouth that I had ever had. A few hours after having the filling installed, I felt a sore throat coming on. On January 21, I awoke from my sleep, not feeling well. Earlier in the day I had been drinking cider. I have shivering and chills, I wrote. What is it about the cider that is poisoning me? I felt nervous and shaky and had a muddy taste in my mouth. I continued to be awakened at night periodically with chills and shivering throughout the next three months despite the fact that I dressed warmly and slept under numerous blankets. I had no virus. I had a gut feeling that I was being poisoned.

March 3rd I recorded being seriously chilled while being out for just a little while in a heavy, wet snowstorm. I got so shaky and cold, and my heart beat so heavily and rapidly, that I turned around and went home. Even after warming up with a hot tea, I still felt sick and shaken. This happened again on March 17, a mild day (40 degrees at 11 a.m.). I got so cold and shaky, even though I was bundled up, I thought I would faint. Why couldn't I take the cold anymore?

A trip to the doctor in February had yielded nothing, so I was on my own to figure this puzzle out. My life was a model of healthy habits: organic food, good attitude, meaningful work, and (prior to January) enough sleeping time. I scanned books in the health section of libraries and bookstores. Finally in April 1985 I came across an article about mercury in dental amalgam and how it affects the immune system. Suddenly it flashed in my mind that all my new health woes began only after my first ever amalgam filling had been placed in January. I called my dentist and, upon my insistence, he replaced my amalgam filling with a composite (plastic) filling on May 6.

Although I didn't expect to feel better immediately, I did. After that same day I felt as though a burden had been lifted from me, as though the sun shone brighter and life was easier. The shivering and the feeling of being poisoned disappeared immediately and have not returned. I regained my endurance and, in all the winters since 1985, I've handled the cold well. It is disappointing to me that neither my doctor nor my dentist had much curiosity about my case.

---

12. Chemicals and Mental Deterioration

I am 38 years old and I have had silver fillings in my mouth since I was a child, but they had no noticeable effect on me until my early thirties. At age 30 I became allergic to molds, dust and yeast and became increasingly sensitive to chemicals. Chemicals affect you mentally as a person would be affected who had environmental illness. This includes disorientation and lack of concentration.

I was diagnosed with a systemic yeast infection by an environmental allergist in Wisconsin. Systemic yeast infection includes a condition known as candidacies. I learned from an acquaintance that mercury in my fillings could be the cause of my symptoms.

After learning that amalgam fillings contain approximately 50% mercury and that it leaks out, I asked a cooperative dentist to remove my fillings. He removed all of my silver fillings and replaced them with another material that did not contain mercury. Now I feel an increased ability to cope and a greater calmness. My strength is growing with each passing day.

I have no doubt that so-called silver fillings were the cause of my illness. Dentists should be required to tell patients that silver fittings contain mercury.

---

13. Anger-Headaches-Depression-Reading

I had good health all my life until about ten years ago. By1986 when

I got married I had 13 fillings and two nickel crowns. Nickel is not as toxic as mercury, but it is toxic. About 1986, I began to get headaches, I was tired all the time, I was anxious, I had fits of anger, and I was always picking fights with my wife. I would get headaches two or three times a week, usually in the afternoon. They were intense, throbbing headaches.

By 1989 or 1990 I had developed a constant sore throat. The throat was so sore it was hard to swallow. By this time I was always catching colds, but doctors couldn't find any infection.

My mother and sister saw the stress in my relationship with my wife and in 1989 they sent me a copy of *Dentistry Today*. It had an article saying that the Environmental Protection Agency had declared dental amalgam a hazardous waste. Through Dr. Huggins' clinic in Colorado, I found Dr. Gary Jacobson. At my request, Dr. Jacobson removed 13 amalgam fillings in four visits in the fall of 1990. After half my fillings were removed, I felt better. I felt calmer immediately. After the last of my fillings were taken out, I felt like a huge burden had been lifted. Within a week of the removal of my last filling, my headaches went away. My outlook on life has really changed. I no longer fight with my wife. I believe the removal of my fillings saved our marriage.

I also understand books better. I never read much before because reading wasn't easy. I had trouble comprehending and remembering what I had read. Now I have much more confidence in my ability to read and to talk about what I've learned.

I don't understand why I learned about mercury in fillings from my family instead of from my dentist. I think dentists should be required to tell patients silver fillings contain mercury.

---

14. Memory Problems

In my case, the improvement was tremendous. In fact, the removal of my amalgams may have saved my life.

I can divide my health history roughly into four parts: age 0 to 8 or 9 when I got my first fillings; age 8 or 9 to age 37 during which my health deteriorated steadily; age 37 to 43 during which time I was so sick I became disabled; life since age 43, the age at which I had my fillings removed.

The first signs of what would be 30+ years of declining health appeared shortly after I got my first amalgams at age 8 or 9. Soon after receiving those fillings, I suffered chronic bouts of strep throat, sinusitis accompanied by severe headaches, and tonsillitis. I lived in fear of the next sinus headache where the pain would be blinding and I would have to endure another trip to the doctor for a shot of penicillin. My interpretation of these symptoms today is that the mercury from my fillings quickly weakened my young immune system and made me vulnerable to throat and sinus infections.

Despite these health problems, I was an exceptional student during my grade-school years. My IQ tests were higher than those of my five siblings, all of whom are very intelligent college graduates who today are successful professionals. In fact, I was so far ahead of my classmates that my school wanted me to skip third or fourth grade. But my parents declined to do that so as not to place me in the same class as an older sister.

But my academic performance deteriorated steadily during my junior and senior high school years due to chronic pain in my brain and the gradual destruction of my ability to concentrate. In senior high I struggled to make the honor rolls, which I used to lead. By the time I entered college I couldn't concentrate on anything. Good study habits became so elusive by my sophomore year that I decided to drop out, shortly before I would have flunked out. In ten years I went from an exceptional student to a college dropout who watched his dreams evaporate.

Instead of becoming a wildlife biologist and a journalist, I took a job in a polluted factory after dropping out of college. From age 25 to 31, I worked as firefighter, a job I enjoyed. But I had to take a medical retirement from that job at age 32 because the cartilage in my right knee had degenerated so bad I could not pass the physical, despite three operations on that knee. The knee did not deteriorate because of a specific injury. It deteriorated just like my overall health—gradually, continuously, and for no apparent reason. I recall telling my wife and friends around my 30th birthday that I felt like I had suddenly aged 20 years.

My health fell apart in 1986. Another attack of stomach pain led to my appendectomy. I was taking antibiotics almost constantly for throat and urinary infections. I was also taking over-the-counter medication constantly to combat pain in the joints and muscles throughout my body. Until 1992, when I got my fillings removed, I also suffered from allergies, asthma, infected sinuses, bronchitis, jaw, neck and chest pain, giardiasis (an intestinal infection), and depression. In the final year and a half prior to getting my amalgams removed, I had become what I can best term a zombie. My brain just wouldn't do anything and my body felt like it weighed a thousand pounds. With the advice of my doctors and my wife, I decided to apply for Social Security benefits because then I could get my medical bills paid and provide my family some desperately needed income. I was assigned an advocate and we began the arduous application process, a process I was told would take over a year. I didn't believe I would live that long. I encountered so many roadblocks that I eventually gave up trying to get Social Security benefits and prayed for a miracle. The miracle came eventually, but not before I had to declare bankruptcy under the weight of my medical bills.

In early 1992 a chiropractor friend of mine called me to say he thought I might have mercury poisoning. He loaned me a copy of *It's All in Your Head* by Dr. Huggins, a mercury-free dentist in Colorado. Through the Huggins clinic I got Dr. Gary Jacobson's phone number. Dr. Jacobson, at my request, removed my amalgams in four sittings in August 1992. I experienced an immediate clearing of my mind after the last session.[96] The morning after my final session, I awoke and trekked to the bathroom. It wasn't until after I was in the bathroom that I realized I had simply popped out of bed and walked like a normal man. I hadn't used the wall and furniture to brace myself and help myself along. My energy was much improved. I even made 24 tomato cages out of used hog wire that day.

Four months later I landed a job with one of the Midwest's largest heart catheter companies, a job that required concentration and an ability to synthesize complex information. My job was to read patent literature and technical medical articles on new products. The number-two guy in the entire corporation told me that I did it very well for the six months our project lasted. I have worked steadily at a variety of other jobs since my patent research job ended.

I no longer suffer from chronic infections and stiffness. I still have occasional bouts of depression that has no apparent trigger other than exercise, which may cause my body to release mercury into my blood stream. My concentration and creativity have improved immensely, but have yet to return to levels I enjoyed decades ago. I have no doubt that mercury from my fillings caused the long history of suffering I have just described.

---

15. Partial Recovery from ALS

I am a female physical education instructor. I grew up on farms in South Dakota and California where I was exposed to a lot of mercury in fungicides. But I was basically pretty healthy until age 17 when I had eight to ten silver fillings placed. From then on I tired more easily and needed more sleep than other people. I also began to get a chronic sore throat. At age 24 I had another eight to ten fillings placed. Within five years I was getting frequent sinus infections and headaches. Within

96 This does happen on occasion, but getting well again usually takes a lot of hard work.

ten years, by which time I was in my mid-thirties, I started to have real bad heat intolerance. I would go out to mow the lawn and right away I would feel weak and get a headache and have to go inside.

During the winter of 1993-94, my health began to deteriorate. My sore throat got worse. My feet started falling asleep and feeling numb and tingly. My right hand got weaker. I couldn't squeeze a fingernail clipper or squeeze a needle into basketballs and footballs to inflate them. I developed pain in my liver, chest and kidneys, as well as muscle dances under my skin in my arms.

In May 1994, I visited a physician at the Minneapolis Clinic of Neurology. He diagnosed me with ALS. Although he mentioned that mercury is sometimes the cause of ALS, he said nothing about mercury from fillings as a possible cause of mercury poisoning. At that time I had no idea my amalgams contained mercury. I learned that by listening to two dentists, Dr. Gary Jacobson and Dr. Huggins, on WCCO Radio on August 16, 1994. I immediately set up an appointment with Dr. Huggins. (Dr. Jacobson could not see me immediately.) On the trip out to Colorado Springs, where Dr. Huggins practiced at the time, I had to lie down in the car most of the way. After Dr. Huggins removed 18 silver fillings, I immediately had more energy and the organ pain went away. On the trip back to Minnesota I didn't lie down once.

Unfortunately, my neurological signs including muscle weakness and spasms did not improve. They did, however, stop getting worse for three months after getting my fillings removed. Since November 1994, my muscles have gotten weaker. But I have no doubt that the removal of my fillings improved my health. If I had not removed my fillings, I am sure I would have had kidney or liver failure by now. I wish the dentist who put fillings in my mouth when I was 17 had told me the fillings contained mercury.

16. Recovered Thought Process

My son recovered from arthritis, and I recovered from osteoporosis, when we had our fillings removed. At age 22, Stephen received a diagnosis of arthritis from a Mayo Clinic physician. The arthritis was so severe that Stephen, a professional organist, could no longer perform. By age 23 he was confined to a bed and a wheel chair. His Mayo Clinic doctor said he would never get out of the wheel chair. In the final six months prior to getting his filings removed, Stephen's mind was so clouded he couldn't read.

Through a Nevada clinic, we learned about Dr. Huggins, a mercury-free dentist in Colorado. In May 1989 my son and I both had our fillings removed by Dr. Huggins. Within a year Stephen was performing again. In 1994 he played at the Notre Dame Cathedral.

And now, I will share my own story with you. I was diagnosed with osteoporosis at the Mayo Clinic in 1984 at age 52. My osteoporosis disappeared after getting my fillings removed in 1989. You have defied all the research, said a physician at the Mayo Clinic. I can also think more clearly and my husband says I am less irritable.

17. Short-term Memory Loss, Depression, Slurred Speech and MS

For years I was in denial, not believing that I was as bad as I was. Things were pretty rough for a long time, but they are getting better now after taking the alternative healing approach. I've been told that this alternative stuff is anecdotal and only works because I've made up my mind that it's going to. That's hogwash! All the years I was going to medical doctors and taking their prescription drugs, I was trying to will myself well. I wasn't able to do it...at least not until I helped my body help itself with the holistic approach. I was so skeptical that I almost didn't try it. I didn't think it would work, but I was desperate.

I only wish I had known about holistic healing 12 years ago when I first started having symptoms. But I know it now, and I plan to keep on doing it. What we didn't realize back then was that medical doctors only treat the symptoms of MS, not the cause.They will tell you there is no known cause and no known cure. They only give you prescription medications, which treat the symptoms, and do nothing for the cause.

I owe so much to my wonderful husband who just wouldn't take no for an answer. Thank you, Duncan, for all your time and efforts researching the Internet, for all the errands and shopping that you've done single-handedly for so many years now, for not giving up on me when the medical doctors did. Thank you for loving me. I love you.

---

18. My Progress in Multiple Sclerosis after Amalgam Removal

I am a 53-year-old housewife who was diagnosed with MS in January 1985. My symptoms varied and fluctuated but included balancing problems, trouble walking, legs felt very heavy, knees buckling, frequent falls, muscle spasms in legs, tremors in hands, loss of appetite, recurring nausea, severe constipation, incontinence—both bladder and bowel, chronic bladder and kidney infections, chronic fatigue, pain in hands, stinging and burning/electric shock sensation in my feet and legs, severe depression, mood swings, temporary partial paralysis in legs, short term memory loss, loss of concentration, confusion, slurred speech, difficulty in making even simple decisions.

My treatments included countless prescription medications, IV steroids (methylprednisolone) and chemotherapy (a cytotoxin). For 9 years I followed medical doctors' advice and only continued to get worse.

We had seen the "60 Minutes" report about the dangers of mercury poisoning from mercury amalgam (silver) dental fillings that aired in December 1990 and the possibility of a link between mercury poisoning and chronic degenerative diseases. We started checking into that possibility and bought a copy of the book *It's All In Your Head* by Dr. Huggins. It sounded pretty far-fetched to us and pretty unbelievable. So we asked my neurologist and dentist about it. They both laughed and told us that it was a hoax and said there was nothing to it. Both of them said that amalgam removal would be a waste of time and money. We asked my neurologist if nutrition would help. He said it probably wouldn't help, but it wouldn't hurt. So try it if you want to. We continued listening to the doctors for a few more years. Then finally my neurologist told me he had done all he could do for me and for me to go home and if I got worse, call him. We were not satisfied with that suggestion! My husband felt there must be something we could do.

In April 1994 I went to a chiropractor/nutritionist who started me on juicing fresh organic fruits and vegetables and taking herbal colon cleansers.

My nausea cleared up and my appetite began to improve in less than a week. I no longer needed my daily anti-nausea medication. My constipation of six years was gone in less than two weeks. My then-current neurologist had been telling me constipation is just part of having MS. Learn to live with it and take a laxative of your choice. Well, I learned I didn't have to live with it. When my appetite came back, my strength soon began to improve.

When we asked my nutritionist about amalgams, he immediately said that it would be necessary to get them out in order to totally detoxify my body. This was further reinforced by an organization named DAMS (Dental Amalgam Mercury Syndromes). They published a book, *Defense Against Mystery Syndromes*, with many first-hand personal stories about different degenerative diseases that were cured or greatly improved by removal of dental mercury amalgam fillings.

We searched the web and found an incredible amount of information on amalgams. Since I had about 14 fillings, we decided to have them replaced. We weren't sure amalgam removal would work, but I was desperate and felt I had to give it a try. I had my amalgams replaced with non-toxic composites in November 1994.

At first I was disappointed and depressed that there was no immediate change, except for the fact that I was able to quit taking all of my prescription medications in December 1994 and did not notice any bad effects from doing so. Prior to this I had tried to cut down on my medications, but was unable to. As recommended by Dr. Huggins, three months after we got back, I took five EDTA chelation treatments to remove the mercury poison that had accumulated in my body over the years. He had explained how mercury vapor is released from the amalgams as you chew and that it accumulates in your cells, tissues and organs. Not feeling any different after five chelation treatments, we decided not to continue with them. We didn't realize at that time just how significant they could be. In the meantime I kept on juicing and watching my diet.

Then about 6 or 8 months later we started noticing subtle improvements. Looking back, we realized that as the nausea had faded away, my appetite improved. As my appetite improved, my strength started coming back, and my knees quit buckling. I quit falling and was soon able to walk some without holding on to anything. Then we noticed that the tremors, slurred speech, and short-term memory loss had gone. I've had only one bladder infection in the past three years and I was able to cure it without antibiotics. My immune system is beginning to work again. I used GranActin from the Health Food Store and added lots of cranberries in my juices. Prior to amalgam removal I was having bladder infections almost continuously. I have more energy and no longer need to take daily naps. When I realized what was happening, we both got very excited and happy. With the arrival of new hope for recovery, I lost my depression and started acting happy and smiling again for the first time in years. The change was so slow and gradual that we didn't notice it was happening for a while.

In trying to get even better, I began the Gerson Therapy at home in February 1996. This is an intensive nutrition and detoxification treatment for cancer, heart disease, diabetes, arthritis, and other chronic degenerative diseases, including MS. It consists of flooding your body with pure nutrition and live enzymes (building blocks to help the body assimilate the nutrients) by drinking lots of fresh organic vegetable and fruit juices, and detoxifying your body from all the years of accumulated toxins.

On this program, you eat only fresh fruits and vegetables, nothing from a can, box or jar. You eat nothing with preservatives, sugar, salt, flour, or anything that has had insecticide on it. For water, you drink only purified water—no chlorine or fluoride is allowed. No insecticides are to be used inside the house. When needed, use a fly swatter. No hair coloring, makeup or hair spray. All toxins are to be eliminated. To allow the body to heal itself, it needs detoxification and the right nutrients for fuel. It's a shame that what we were taught as kids to be good nutrition really isn't. Also, you can't cook in aluminum or Teflon-coated cookware. Aluminum is to be strictly avoided, including alum, baking powder and deodorants made with aluminum.

I took more chelation treatments until I had a total of 25. I continue to improve. Last summer I even got my driver's license after not driving for 9 years. I still have problems. Stinging and burning pain in my feet and legs, although more tolerable now, is still with me. But it doesn't put me under like it used to. I still ride my electric scooter, but probably only about 1/2 as much now as I did three years ago. I can walk farther from my scooter now. However, the more I walk, the more it hurts. Since amalgam removal and change in diet, ALL my symptoms are either IMPROVED or GONE! The pain is my worst problem now, but it is nothing like it used to be.

Four years before we were ready to listen, a friend of ours had tried to tell us about the dangers of amalgams. It took me that much longer of going downhill and getting worse before my husband and I gave up on the medical profession and began listening to our friend. He had been through amalgam removal, chelation and the Gerson Therapy and had cured his Chronic Fatigue Syndrome.

For the past 4 years since trying alternative healing methods, I have continued to get better. Please read my story on our web site at http://cust2.iamerica.net1mirage/idstory.htm. I am so glad we finally decided to stop listening to my neurologist. I only wish we had done this sooner. I truly believe I would not have gotten as bad as I did and would have recovered 100% by now.

---

19. "60 Minutes" Recovery Stories

Fay Doris: Dr. Vimy took a mercury test of the mercury vapor in my mouth, and at that point it was the highest of anybody he'd tested. I had ten teeth with massive mercury fillings in them, and uh, as he said at the time, if I was a building I would have been condemned (laugh), the reading was so high!

Morley Safer: Fay Doris and her husband are patients of Dr. Vimy. She was crippled by arthritis, suffered from fatigue, colitis, and memory loss. Her Dr. told her back in 1985 at the age of 35 that within 6 months she'd be confined to a wheelchair. After reading about a connection between mercury and arthritis, Dave Doris talked to Dr. Vimy about removing his wife's fillings.

Dave Doris: And I said, go ahead and do it, what have we got to lose. The prognosis is she's going to be in a wheelchair by Christmas for the rest of her life, which was scary for me.

Fay Doris: I was mercury free by, I think by the 21st of August of that year, and 3, within 3 weeks later I didn't have to use a cane, and all my symptoms started going away. I had more energy, my tremor stopped in my hands, I could do things again, it was just marvelous.

Dave Doris: And noticeably the swelling in the joints of her hands, uh, started to go down, but the biggest thing was, it wasn't painful on her feet to walk.

Safer: And have, have any of those symptoms returned?

Fay Doris: On the whole, I'd say 95% of it is gone away.

(Cut to Dr. Vimy)

Vimy: That's clinical evidence. That's not scientific evidence, but clinical evidence is where science has to start. Science starts with observation.

Safer: The kind of evidence Dr. Vimy is talking about is what scientists call anecdotal, reports of recoveries that have not been monitored under strict laboratory conditions. There are thousands of anecdotal stories, all over Europe and the United States. A group in Illinois reported relief from symptoms of manic depression, chronic fatigue, and migraine headaches, from multiple sclerosis and anemia.

(Cut to Nancy Yost interview)

Safer: Last May, Nancy Yost, from San Jose, was told by her doctors that she had multiple sclerosis. It was confirmed by Magnetic Resonance Imaging, an MRI scan, incurable. She'd worked in the dental industry, and heard reports that some patients showed improvement after having amalgam fillings removed.

Yost: And I was cautioned by the doctors always: You've got your hopes too high, get real here (laugh). If you are better, it's going to be a long period.

Safer: Ohhhh. As a last resort, she had her five amalgam fillings taken out. She left the dentist's office using a cane and leaning heavily on the arm of a friend.

Yost: The next morning, when I was presented to my physician, I threw my cane at him, and said look!

Safer: It was that quick?

Yost: It was that quick.

Safer: What did your doctor say?

Yost: Well, he was incredulous. He knew it would be a benefit, but no one expected it would be instantaneous, or so dramatic. My voice came back; my ability to walk and hold a pencil came back. It was there! That night, I ended up going to dinner in San Francisco and actually dancing 2 dances. And I hadn't been walking since May (laugh)!

Safer: Next day.

Yost: Friday evening, the next day.

Safer: Are there any lingering effects?

Yost: Yes. There are lingering effects if I get overtired, or cold, or under a great deal of stress.

(Cut to Dr. Heber Simmons, president of the ADA)

Simmons: The National Multiple Sclerosis Society states that this is a cruel hoax on these people, to take the fillings out in hopes that it's going to cure the MS, and it does not happen in those cases, it simply does not happen.

Yost: I think it's a rather strange position to take, because according to all the doctors I talked to, they said multiple sclerosis has no....no known cause, and there is no known cure. Well, if we don't know what causes it, why not look at possibilities? Might it be mercury poisoning? They have no better answer!

Safer: There's no suggestion that all MS patients will recover if their fillings are removed. But there are enough recoveries or partial recoveries to raise questions. There are alternatives to amalgams. Composites like Dr. Vimy's placing in this patient's mouth, porcelain and gold. They're all more expensive than amalgam, and except for gold, not as durable. Amalgams are also easier for dentists to use.

While the ADA publicly advocates the safety of amalgam, it cautions dentists to use a no-touch technique when handling the material, and to store the scrap, the leftovers that have not gone into a patient's mouth, under liquid in a tightly closed container.

(Cut to Dr. Heber Simmons, ADA)

Safer: If it's so volatile, so dangerous in a dentist's hands, how on earth can it be safe in our mouths?

Simmons: Morley, you've got to understand, uh, how amalgam really works. If it's in a free form, the mercury that is in amalgam is dangerous. But it, when it forms with the copper, the tin, the zinc, and the silver that, that make up the amalgam filling, it becomes a stable compound at that time. Once it is mixed and placed in a patient's mouth, it is a stable compound and it does not constitute a risk.

Safer: Once it hardens......

Simmons: Correct.

Safer: It's safe.

Simmons: Right.

Safer: What do you do with your scrap amalgam?

Simmons: What we do in our own practice is we keep it in a jar that has glycerin in the jar, we put the scrap in there—put a top on it, so it is not exposed in any way. It's in an airtight jar all the time.

Safer: Why, given that...?

Simmons: That is the recommended way of taking care of it in a dental office. That's what's been recommended by the scientists, so that's the way we do it.

Safer: But if it's so perfectly safe in this combined state.......

Simmons: But Morley, you've got to understand when we, uh, when we're saving this stuff, we, we've got a big jar of it. You've got to realize I'm in that office five days a week, with this material. I do not want to go in there with an open container like that. I want to be as safe as I can.

(Cut to Dr. Joel Berger interview)

Safer: The ADA is adamant that mercury in a patient's mouth is safe. So adamant that in 1986 it changed its code of ethics. It became a violation of that code for any dentist to recommend the removal of amalgam because of mercury. Almost immediately Dr. Joel Berger, a visible and vocal anti-amalgam dentist, was charged with fraud by the New York State dental authorities. The ADA provided an expert witness to testify against him. His license was revoked.

Berger: I never told a patient that they would get healthier or better. I told them that we could remove a known risk, a poison, a toxin, and a carcinogen, from their bodies if they eliminate the source of mercury from their mouths. It was their risk decision to do it or not to do it.

Dr. Vimy: Dr. Joel Berger should never have lost his, uh, dental license. He was a very conservative dentist. You couldn't even consider him a fringe dentist. Dr, Vimy testified as a scientific expert for Joel Berger. He says the change in the code of ethics has had a profound effect.

Vimy: The effect has been that it's really, in the United States, taken away the constitutional rights of dentists and the rights of patients. They have, they no longer have freedom of choice, and they no longer have freedom of expression. A dentist can no longer say that he is against dental amalgam, so it's a fear tactic; it's a witch-hunt.

(Cut to Dr. Simmons, ADA)

Simmons: But I can tell you that we are not on a witch-hunt. That I personally am not. That's a personal choice that the dentist has to make.

Safer: Why did you change the code of ethics regarding amalgams?

Simmons: Because it has not been proven that taking amalgams out will help any of these conditions. And there were people that were taking amalgams out, saying that that was going to help MS and other conditions. It has never been scientifically proven that this will happen.

(Cut to Dr. Murray Vimy)

Safer: What's the position of the Canadian Dental Association?

Vimy: Exactly the same. The Americans sneeze, the Canadians bring their Kleenex. So they have changed their code of ethics too.

(Cut to Dr. Simmons)

Safer: How do you account for those people whose health has improved after the removal of amalgam fillings?

Simmons: I would have to say that it was anecdotal. I'm delighted that the people are better.

(Cut to Dr. Alfred Zamm interview)

Zamm: The word anecdote doesn't mean it's not true. It means it's an observed clinical observation by a clinician, and that's my job. I'm a clinician. And I saw the patient got better, what am I supposed to do, report that he didn't get better?

Safer: Dr. Alfred Zamm is an allergist and dermatologist in Kingston, New York. He's reported that hundreds of his patients have recovered from a variety of diseases after having fillings removed. He's in the process of filing those cases with the Food and Drug Administration. One case is a 32-year-old woman who was crippled by arthritis.

Zamm: And I had her seen by a board-certified rheumatologist who's really a good physician, he really knows what he's doing. And he said, "there's a limit to what I can do" and he gave her some anti-inflammatory drugs and aspirin, and so forth.

Safer: Dr. Zamm arranged for her fillings to be removed. Within a month, she was no longer on crutches. The rheumatologist was astounded. Not only was her arthritis better, but also you could see she looked like a different person. She was healthy. She no longer was poisoned.

(Cut to Dr. Simmons, ADA)

Safer: Do you totally dismiss the anecdotal evidence?

Simmons: No, I do not totally dismiss it. But I just say on the basis of the facts that we have today, they're insignificant. They're clinically insignificant.

Zamm: How could they know that? Do they examine the patient 3 or 6 months later? How many dentists have done a rectal on you (just to be ridiculous). They don't know anything about you!

Simmons: You've got to remember, we're, we're looking at, at, really a long time use. You know there have only been 50 cases reported in the literature of amalgam allergy, of true allergy to amalgam in the last 85 years.

Zamm: That's an obfuscating statement. They use the word allergic. It's not allergy. It's poisoning of critical immune processes. If someone dies of cancer, and you ask the specialist "why does he have cancer?" He says, "I don't know." If someone dies of heart disease, "why did this one get heart disease and the other one didn't?" "I don't know." There are a lot of things we don't know. But I do know that it's not safe to put something in somebody's mouth that has a question.

Safer: Dr. Zamm has charted symptoms of diseases, patients who've had fillings removed, and the results. He points to Joe Seveski as a prime example. For years, he suffered with allergies to certain foods. Then 5 years ago, he began getting serious infections. It went on for 4 years.

Zamm: I sent him to a board-certified internist who was a specialist in blood disease who could find nothing.

Safer: Finally Dr. Zamm had Joe's fillings removed. Within a month the infections were gone.

Zamm: His unexplained rashes of 20 years had disappeared. Now he can eat foods that he couldn't eat before. His immune system is working again.

Safer: Nothing wrong with his blood?

Zamm: Board-certified specialist could not find a thing.

Safer: No other change in his environment that could account for this?

Zamm: Zero, no change whatsoever. We're just arguing here, or discussing, whether a poison is a poison. It's a bizarre conversation, you know, when you think about it. To try to justify if a poison is a poison.

Safer: If the mercury in amalgam fillings is as poisonous as you say it is, why hasn't the medical community jumped on it and banned it?

Zamm: Goodman and Gilman is the Bible of Pharmacology. When you go to medical school, you use Goodman and Gilman. According to Goodman and Gilman, there have been epidemics of mercury poisoning that were misdiagnosed for years. The reason for the tragic delays, says this textbook, include vagueness of early clinical signs and the medical profession's unfamiliarity with the disease.

This author could write dozens of similar recovery stories but this chapter might need to be two inches thick. It would take more stress, time and expenditure than I am willing to pay to collect those stories and verify their authenticity. In addition, most of my friends who suffered from chronic low-level mercurial poisoning prefer not to talk about their ordeal. Our stories are too painful to relive by the telling. Perhaps I should put it this way: before we disbanded ADAMS (A Dental Amalgam Mercury Syndrome Group) there were at least 400 dues-paying members in the greater Seattle area. All of us have simi-

lar stories. What we all need is closure, not to reopen old wounds. For the ADA to say tens of thousands of similar stories around the world are only anecdotal evidence, that mercury does not cause short-term memory loss (and many other diseases), is an insult to our intelligence.

Epilogue

I hadn't laughed in two years. I was depressed and burnt out. I couldn't work anymore. We'd lost our home and were broke. I wasn't able to support those who depended upon me. I had to crawl up the stairs and rest a couple of times between landings. My despicable behavior and hostility decimated our entire family. I would have preferred to die than cause so much trouble and heartache.

Then in June of 1983 I was diagnosed with Alzheimer's disease at St. Peter Hospital at Olympia, Washington. Three other physicians confirmed the diagnosis. I visited our state mental hospital's Alzheimer's ward at Tacoma, Washington, and performed a Shakespearean act keeping my composure. I was terrorized by the end stages of the Alzheimer's and would have rather been shot a hundred times than die that way. Eventually I realized that I wasn't going to improve and would have to go through the end stages of the disease process, so I prayed: Lord, let me die! One morning I was sitting in a chair and staring at my shoes, feeling miserable. Louise's Bible was near and I picked it up and started reading Job. I understood the meaning of what I read but could not remember the gist of the sentence for more than four inches of print. My long-term memory seemed to recall Job suffered terribly and through all of his torment that Job continued to praise God. Suddenly I broke out laughing as if Bob Hope told a hilarious joke and said, "Satan, you're going to lose because I'm going to praise Jesus with my dying breath." In that instant I quit worrying about what might or might not happen. It seemed Jesus was sitting in the chair beside me. Of course I could not see him. But he was there and I said, "Jesus, if I have to die this death, at least through me let the cure for Alzheimer's disease be found." We had a lovely new apartment that was really tight. There were no drafts. The next day a soft gentle breeze blew through a hallway that I knew was the Holy Spirit.

Naively, I tied to scribble notes that I hoped might point researchers to some clue that might help other Alzheimer's sufferers before my thought process completely evaporated, but writing is a cerebral-motor function and no one, not even my wife who is a registered pharmacist accustomed to reading doctor's prescriptions, could decipher my scrawl. Louise purchased a Kaypro computer, and the notes that I hoped might point neurologists toward a breakthrough for Alzheimer's disease turned into my first book, *Beating Alzheimer's*. In those days there was no Internet. Research was restricted to medical journals and university medical libraries. It was easier to cover-up medical bloopers. We allowed the informed to do our thinking for us. The Internet has changed all that. There is so much solid evidence that the ADA continues to cover up—that they have poisoned a minimum of 200,000,000 American citizens—available from unimpeachable sources on the Internet, the ADA publishes disinformation to stem the tide. However, there are more than a dozen MSDS sheets that mimic Caulk's revelations in Section 2 of this book on the Internet.

It is not a case of waiting until you become ill to get around to reading this book. Knowing these things can prevent millions of our population from suffering dozens of gut-wrenching chronic diseases. If you learn these things, it could save the reader hundreds of thousands of dollars in lost income and unnecessary medical expenses. And, if you read this message in time, provided you are a saver and an investor, it will allow your family to keep your economic goals intact so your spouse can live out his or her twilight years in health and comfort.

This paragraph is my closure. It completes the promise that I made to the Lord 19 years ago. I hope He is pleased and that the reader is also pleased. "May the road rise to meet you. May the wind always be at your back. May the rain fall soft upon your fields. Until we meet again, may the Lord hold you in the hollow of His hand."

Chronic Low-Level Mercurial Poisoning and Chronic Disease

This section of the book is designed to present to health professionals scientific evidence concerning the toxicity of mercury. For information about root canals, cavitations and focal infections, *see Chapter 2 and Appendix XIII.*

Material Safety Data Sheets

A Material Safety Data Sheet (MSDS) reflects the hazards of working with a material in an occupational fashion. For example, an MSDS for paint is not highly pertinent to someone who uses a can of paint once a year, but is extremely important to someone who does this in a confined space 40 hours a week.

Dentsply Caulk[97] (in business since 1899) is one of the world's foremost manufacturers of dental amalgam. This, in part, is an MSDS sheet Caulk posted on the Internet April 1997. USA Today reported in February 1998 that the ADA had Caulk remove the MSDS Sheet from their Web Page because dental patients found the report too upsetting (too revealing-author).

97 Dentsply Caulk, 38 West Clarke Avenue, Milford, DE 19963-0359.

Dentsply Caulk
MSDS

...Chronic Inhalation of mercury vapor over a long period may cause depression or despondency, resentment of criticism, irritability or excitability, headache, fatigue, insomnia, hallucinations, loss of memory and mental deterioration may occur. Concentrations as low as 0.03 mg/m 3 have induced psychiatric symptoms in humans. ...Mercury is excreted in breast milk...

Weiss Instruments
MSDS

...Paralysis, loss of memory, chronic renal[98] disease, gum disease, constriction of the visual field and strong disinclination to work, mental fatigue, irritability, excitability, headaches, digestive disturbance, timidity. . . and the need for an unusual amount of dental work. ...People with chronic disease or poor health should be excluded from mercury exposure.

---

98 ...Significantly increased risks for chronic renal failure (CRF) were found for exposure to lead, copper, chromium, tin, mercury, welding fumes, silicon compounds, grain dusts, and oxygenated hydrocarbons. The frequency of exposure to these agents was higher in CRF patients with diabetic nephropathy, renal vascular disease, and glomerulonephritis. Mean blood lead concentrations were significantly higher in the cases than in the controls. The authors conclude that the study confirms previously identified risk factors for CRF such as heavy metal exposures and suggest that some new exposures, e.g., grain dust, might increase the risk.....Lancet, 346(8966): 1995
(*Grain farmers pour mercury into open troughs along the outside bottom of grain elevators to eliminate pests. They spray mercury into the top of grain elevators to poison flying insects and birds. All grain silos are contaminated with mercury-author.*)

Kerr: Division of Sybron Corp MSDS

...Special Hazard Precautions: Eating or smoking should not be permitted in areas where mercury is handled or stored.

Environmental Resource Associates MSDS Health Hazards, Acute and Chronic:

Poison ...May cause GI tract perforations[99] and pulmonary edema ...

Chronic exposure through any route can produce central nervous system damage. May cause muscle tremor, personality and behavior changes, memory loss, and metallic taste, loosening of the teeth, digestive disorders, skin rashes, brain and kidney damage....

Environmental Chemicals Data and Information Network ECDIN Human Health Effects of Mercury

...The target organ is the central nervous system. The pronounced clinical symptoms are evident changes in handwriting, and speech becomes monotonous, syllabized stammering, irritability, and changes in socialness, anxiety and loss of memory. ...May cause birth defects, especially brain damage. Avoid exposure to pregnant women....

Agency for Toxic Substances and Disease Registry (ATSDR) 1999

Toxicological profile for mercury: Atlanta, GA: U.S. Department of Health and Human Services.

---

99 Leaky-Gut Syndrome.

Exposure to mercury occurs from breathing contaminated air, ingesting contaminated water and food, and having dental and medical treatments. Mercury, at high levels, may damage the brain, kidneys, and developing fetus.

How can mercury affect my health?

The nervous system is very sensitive to all forms of mercury. Methylmercury and metallic mercury vapors are more harmful than other forms, because more mercury in these forms reaches the brain. Exposures to high levels of metallic, inorganic, or organic mercury can permanently damage the brain, kidneys, and developing fetus. Effects on brain functioning may result in irritability, shyness, tremors, changes in vision or hearing, and memory problems. Long-term exposure to either organic or inorganic mercury can permanently damage the brain, kidneys, and developing fetuses. ...Breathed metallic mercury vapor may cause greater harm to the brain and developing fetuses . . . Mercury has been shown to cause cancer in humans.[100]

How might I be exposed to mercury?

1. Eating fish or shellfish contaminated with methylmercury.
2. Breathing vapors in air from spills, incinerators, and industries that burn mercury-contaminating fuels.
3. Release of mercury vapor from dental work and medical treatments (including vaccinations).
4. Breathing contaminated air or skin contact during use in the work place (dental health services, chemical and other industries that use mercury).

---

100 Public Health Statement, December 1990.

ATSDR/EPA Priority List for 1997 Top 20 Hazardous Substances

Arsenic

Lead

Mercury, Metallic

Vinyl Chloride etc.

FASEB Dental Mercury is Source of Two-Thirds of Mercury in Population

ABSTRACT:[101] There is a considerable controversy as to whether dental amalgams may cause systemic health effects in humans because they liberate elemental mercury. Most such amalgams contain as much as 50 percent metallic mercury. To determine the influence of dental amalgams on the mercury body burden of humans, we have given volunteers, with and without amalgams in their mouth, the sodium salt of 2, 3-dimercaptopropane-1-sulfonic acid (DMPS), a chelating agent safely[102]used in the Soviet Union and West Germany for a number of years. The diameters of dental amalgams of the subjects were determined to obtain the amalgam score. Administration of 300 mg DMPS by mouth increased the mean urinary mercury excretion of the amalgam group from 0.70 to 17.2 μg and that of the non-amalgam

---

101 Aposhian, H.V., D.C. Bruce, W. Alter, R.C. Dart, K.M. Hurlbut, M.M. Aposhian, "Urinary Mercury after Administration of 2, 3-dimercaptopropane-1-sulfonic acid: Correlation with Dental Amalgam Score" FASEB J. 6: 2472-2476; (1992).

102 It is not safe to use DMPS or any other liquid chelating agent if the patient exhibits symptoms of mental deterioration. All liquid chelating agents dump too much mercury and other metals too quickly that synergistically destroy brain tissue, e.g., the combination of lead and mercury is 100 times more toxic to brain and neurological tissues than either metal by itself.

group from 0.27 to 5.1 μg over a 9-hour period. Two-thirds of the mercury excreted in the urine of those with dental amalgams appears to be derived originally from the mercury vapor released from their amalgams. Linear regression analysis indicated a highly significant positive correlation between the mercury excreted in the urine 2 hours after DMPS administration and the dental amalgam scores. DMPS can be used to increase the urinary excretion of mercury and thus increase the significance and reliability of this measure of mercury exposure or burden, especially in cases of micromercurialism.

The Coors Study

The Coors Study, researched by Dr. Huggins, funded by Adolph Coors Brewing Company, remains unpublished because the ADA has done everything within its power to suppress Dr. Huggins' books and research. In this study Dr. Huggins reports huge amounts of mercury are released during the tooth drilling process. Pieces of dead brain tissue are found in the spinal fluid of dental patients for a 24-hour period after a mercury amalgam filling has been replaced.

In light of this horrifying discovery, for the ADA to deny that mercury—50 percent of a mercury amalgam filling—does not destroy brain tissue is indefensible. No further research should be necessary to discontinue the use of mercury amalgam fillings. Dr. Huggins' research is reproducible and incontrovertible.

Mercury exposure via breast milk: biological trace element research

ABSTRACT:[103] Neonatal uptake of Hg from milk was examined in a

103 Vimy, M.J., Hooper, D.E., King, W.W., Lorscheider, F.L., "Mercury from Maternal 'Silver' Tooth Fillings in Sheep and Human Breast Milk: A Source of Neonatal Exposure." Biological Trace Element Research, 56:143-52, (1997).

pregnant sheep model, where radioactive mercury (Hg203)/silver tooth fillings (amalgam) were newly placed. A crossover experimental design was used in which lactating ewes nursed foster lambs. In a parallel study, the relationship between dental history and breast milk concentration of Hg was also examined.

Results from the animal studies showed that, during pregnancy, a primary fetal site of amalgam Hg concentration is in the liver, and after delivery the neonatal lamb kidney receives additional amalgam Hg from mother's milk.

In lactating women with aged amalgam fillings, increased Hg excretion in breast milk and urine correlated with the number of fillings or Hg vapor concentration levels in mouth air.

It was concluded that Hg originating from maternal amalgam tooth fillings transfers across the placenta to the fetus, across the mammary gland into milk ingested by the newborn and ultimately into neonatal body tissues. Comparisons are made to the U.S. minimal risk level recently established for adult Hg exposure. These findings suggest the placement and removal of "silver" tooth fillings in pregnant and lactating humans will subject the fetus and neonate to unnecessary risk of Hg exposure.

Journal of Neural Transmission

Increased Blood Mercury Levels in Patients with Alzheimer's disease

ABSTRACT:[104] Alzheimer's disease is a common neurodegenerative disorder that leads to dementia and death. In addition to several genetic parameters, various environmental factors may influence the risk

104 C. Hock, G. Drasch, S. Golombowski, F. Muller-Spahn, B. Willershausen-Zonnchen, P. Schwarz, U. Hock, J.H. Growdon, R.M. Nitsch "Increased Blood Mercury Levels in Patients with Alzheimer's Disease" Journal of Neural Transmission, 105: (1998).

of getting AD. In order to test whether blood levels of the heavy metal mercury are increased in AD, we measured blood mercury concentrations in AD patients (n=33), and compared them to age-matched control patients with major depression (MD) (n=45), as well as to an additional control group of patients with various non-psychiatric disorders (n=65). Blood mercury levels were more than two fold higher in AD patients as compared to both control groups (p=0.0005, and p=0.0000, respectively). In early onset AD patients (n=13), blood mercury levels were almost three fold higher as compared to controls (p=0.0002, and p=0.0000, respectively). These increases were unrelated to the patients' dental status. Linear regression analysis of blood mercury concentrations and CSF levels of amyloid B-peptide (AB) revealed a significant correlation of these measures in AD patients (n=15, r=0.7440, p=0.0015, Pearson type of correlation). These results demonstrate elevated blood levels of mercury in AD, and they suggest that this increase of mercury levels is associated with high CSF levels of AB, whereas tau levels were unrelated. Possible explanations of increased blood mercury levels in AD include yet unidentified environmental sources or release from brain tissue with the advance in neuronal death.

Hazardous Chemicals Desk Reference, 4th Edition, by Richard Lewis, Sr.

Dr. Richard Lewis is a chemist with extensive experience in air and industrial pollution measurements, industrial hygiene research and toxicological and chemical information systems. Formerly manager of information systems for the National Institute for Occupational Health and Safety, Dr. Lewis is the author of a number of widely used references including *Sax's Dangerous Properties of Industrial Materials*, 9th Edition, in which he lists every compound of mercury HR: 3. HR: 3 identify the most toxic hazards listed in this reference book.

Long-Term Exposure

Repeated or prolonged exposure to mercury vapor causes effects that develop gradually. The first effects to occur are often fine shaking of the hands, eyelids, lips, tongue, or jaw. Other effects are allergic skin rash, headache, sores in the mouth, sore and swollen gums, loose teeth, insomnia, excess salivation, personality change, irritability, indecision, loss of memory, and intellectual deterioration.

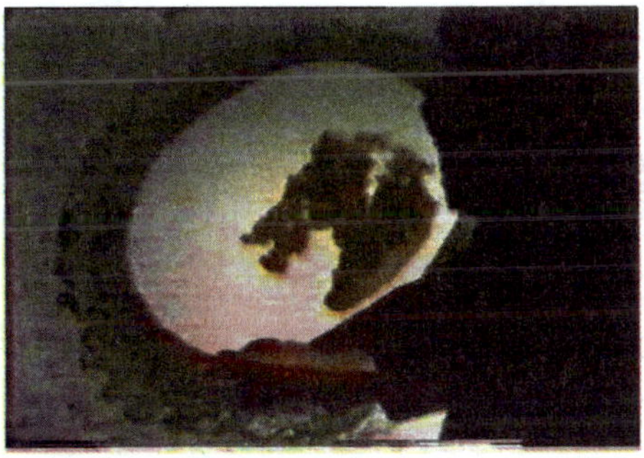

The black ring (arrow) surrounding the artery is mercury, causing atherosclerosis, eventually choking off the artery. The white area is plaque.

"Arteriosclerosis is set in motion when cells lining the arteries are damaged as a result of high blood pressure, smoking, toxic substances in the environemnt, e.g., (mercury poisoning-author), bacteria and other agents. Plaques develop when high-density lipoproteins accumulate at the site of arterial damage and platelets act to form a fibrous cap over this fatty core. Deposits impede or eventually shut off blood flow."
– *Steadman's Medical Dictionary for Health Professionals*

CASRN (EPA Pesticide Database) J.S. EPA IRIS Substance File 7439-97-6

Mercury Vapor Gocs to the Brain

Berlin et al. (1969) exposed rats, rabbits and monkeys to 1 mg/cu.m of mercury vapor for 4 hours and measured the uptake and distribution of mercury in the brain as compared with animals injected intravenously with the same doses of mercury as mercuric salts. Mercury accumulated in the brain following inhalation exposure to metallic mercury vapor at levels that were 10 times higher than those observed following intravenous injection of the same dose of mercury as mercuric salts. These results demonstrate that mercury is taken up by the brain following inhalation of the vapor at higher levels than other forms of mercury and that this occurs in all species studied.

Mercury and the Blood-Brain Barrier

In 1995 the *Journal of Applied Toxicology,* an English academic publication, reported:

"It (mercury) swiftly passes the placental barrier and accumulates in the frontal brain and blood, building up to 30 percent higher red blood cell levels than in the mother."

The Journal of the California Dental Association 12:37 1984.

Recent studies with pregnant women indicate that elemental mercury does cross the hemochorial placenta and incorporates into the fetus. Thus, the placenta, the chorioallantoic membrane, the amniotic membrane, the neonatal blood of women who were exposed to mercury while working in dental offices were found to contain significantly higher levels than in control women with no occupational exposure to mercury.

Dr. Huggins told me, "The fastest way for a woman to get rid of mercury is to have a baby." A newborn infant weighing six to eight pounds at birth accumulates approximately 20 to 30 percent more mercury in its body than its mother. In the first trimester of pregnancy, as the brain and central nervious system is beginning to develop and the fetus is about the size of a quarter, the 20 percent figure is many times more toxic to the diminutive prenatal brain and central nervous system.

Stillbirths and Mercury

Mercury binds to the oxygen-carrying sites on the hemoglobin in the blood. Women with high levels of hemoglobin run an increased risk of stillbirths, offering a possible clue to a tragedy that currently is thought to have no known cause. Dr. Olof Stephansson and colleagues from the Karolinska Institute, Stockholm, Sweden, reported in a study of 1400 pregnant women that those with high hemoglobin levels early in their pregnancy had double the risk of losing their child. *Author's comment: It appears the body produces additional red blood cells to supply enough oxygen-carrying sites for survival. See following citation.*

Journal of the American Medical Association, November 2000.

Levels of hemoglobin, an oxygen-carrying blood protein, can be raised by smoking (and mercury-author), which has also been linked to stillbirths. But this study found no clear association between smoking and hemoglobin and lacked data for the cause of the high levels of hemoglobin.

American Journal of Obstetrics and Gynecology 1982.

A significant association was found between previous stillbirths and mercury levels in both maternal and cord blood.

Journal of Applied Toxicology, 1985.

Mercury in Children's Brains

Concerning the effects of mercury exposure on children as noted at autopsy following their death, the following were noted: (1) the changes in the brain were widespread; the whole cortex was affected, including the frontal lobe. (2) A reduction of brain weight by 26.55 percent was seen.

A Unique Form of Mercury Poisoning

A thorough review of medical literature and U.S. government data indicates (1) that many and perhaps most cases of idiopathic autism, in which an extended period of developmental normalcy is followed by an emergence of symptoms, are induced by early exposure to Hg; (2) that this type of autism represents a unique form of Hg poisoning (HgP); (3) that excessive Hg exposure from vaccine injections is an etiological mechanism for causing the traits of autism; (4) that certain genetic and non-genetic factors establish a predisposition whereby adverse effects occur only in some children; and (5) that vaccinal Hg in thimerosal is causing a heretofore unrecognized mercurial syndrome.

The medical literature also indicates that the characteristics of autism, Alzheimer's and of mercury poisoning (HgP) are strikingly similar. The parallels between the two diseases are so thorough as to suggest, based on total Hg injected into U.S. children, that autism and Alzheimer's are iatrogenic diseases caused by mercury poisoning.

For these children, the exposure route is childhood vaccine, most of which contain thimerosal, a preservative that is 49.6 percent methylmercury by weight.The amount of mercury a typical child under two years receives from vaccinations equates to 237.5 micrograms, or 3.53 x 1017 molecules (353,000,000,000,000,000 molecules). Most such vaccinal Hg may not be excreted and instead migrates to the brain. The total amount injected into infants and toddlers (1) is known to exceed federal safety standards, (2) is officially considered to be a "low" level; whereby (3) only a small percentage of exposed individuals exhibit symptoms of toxicity. In fact, children who develop Hg-related autism are likely to have had a predisposition derived from genetic and non-genetic factors (for example, mercury is excreted from the mother's dental fillings and breast milk-author).

The timings of vaccinal Hg-exposure and its latency period coincide with the emergence of autistic symptoms specific in children. Moreover, excessive mercury has been detected in their urine, hair and blood samples. Parental reports, though limited at the time this book goes to press, indicate significant improvement in symptoms subsequent to heavy-metal chelation therapy.[105]

The HgP phenotype is diverse and depends upon a number of factors—including the type of Hg, route of entry into the body, rate and level of dose, individual genotype, and the age and immune status of the patient. Historically, variation among these factors has caused slightly different manifestations of mercurialism; Mad Hatter's disease, Minamata disease, acrodynia, and industrial exposures provide examples.

The pathology arising from the mercury-related variables involved in autism—intermittent bolus doses of ethylmercury injected into susceptible infants and toddlers—is heretofore undescribed in medical literature. Therefore, in accord with existing HgP data and HgP's ability to induce virtually all the traits defining or associated with autism spectrum disorders, we hypothesize that many and perhaps most cases of autism represent a unique form of mercury poisoning.

This conclusion and its supporting data have important implications for the affected population of autistic children and their families, for other unexplained disorders with symptoms similar to those of heavy metal intoxication, for vaccine content, and for childhood vaccination programs. Due to its high potential for neurotoxicity, thimerosal should be removed immediately from all vaccine products designated for infants and toddlers.

105 Do not use liquid chemical chelation products on children! It would be tantamount to taking the child out of the frying pan and throwing him into the fire. See Chapter 3 and Appendix IV.

National Institutes of Health Reports on the Neurological and Psychiatric Effects of Mercury:

CNS Effects of Mercury:

The most consistent and chronic effects of chronic exposure to elemental mercury are CNS effects, neurological and psychiatric. Common systems include depression, irritability, exaggerated response to stimulation (erethism) and excessive shyness, insomnia, emotional instability, forgetfulness, confusion and vasomotor disturbances.[106]

Goodman and Gilman:
Pharmacological Basis of Therapeutics

Chronic exposure to mercury vapor produces a more insidious form of toxicity that is dominated by neurological effects (Friberg and Vostal 1972). Continued exposure to methylmercury poisoning produces symptoms of depression, irritability, excessive shyness, insomnia, emotional instability, forgetfulness, confusion, increased excitability and renal dysfunction.[107]

British Medical Journal
Chronic Neurobehavioral Effects of Elemental Mercury in Dentists

Neurobehavioral tests were performed by 98 dentists (mean age 32, range 24-49) exposed to elemental mercury vapor and 54 controls

---

106 JAMA Editorial, "Limiting Infant Exposure to Thimerosal in Vaccines and Other Sources of Mercury," Neal A. Halsey, MD, http://www.autism-mercury.com/jama_editorial.htm.

107 Gilman, A.G., L.S. Goodman, and A. Gilman. (Eds.). Goodman and Gilman's The Pharmacological Basis of Therapeutics. 7th Ed. New York: Macmillan Publishing Co., Inc., 1985, p1612. [Peer reviewed.]

(mean age 34, range 23-50) with no history of occupational exposure to mercury. The dentists were exposed to an average personal air concentration time weighted average (TWA) of 0.014 (range 0.0007-0.042) mg/m3 for a mean period of 5.5 (range 0.7-24) years and had a mean blood mercury concentration of 9.8 (range 0.6-57) micrograms/1. In neurobehavioral tests measuring motor speed (finger tapping), visual scanning (trail making), visuomotor coordination and concentration (digit symbol), verbal memory (digit span, logical memory delayed recall), visual memory (visual reproduction, immediate and delayed recall), and visuomotor coordination speed (Bender-Gestalt time), the performance of the dentists was significantly worse than that of the controls. The dentists scored 3.9 to 38.9 percent (mean 13.9 percent) worse in these tests. In trail making, digit span, logical memory delayed recall, visual reproduction, delayed recall, and Bender-Gestalt time, test scores were more than 10 percent poorer. In each of the tests in which significant differences were found and in the block design time, the performance decreased as the exposed dose (product of the TWA of air mercury concentrations and the years of exposure) increased. These results raise the question as to whether the current threshold limit value of 0.050 mg/m3 (TWA) provides adequate protection against adverse effects of mercury.[108]

Journal of the Canadian Dental Association, May 1994; Vol.60, No.5.

In addition, dentists are twice as likely to commit suicide. They have a two times higher divorce rate than the rest of the population, and 20% of all dentists on long-term disability insurance programs have psychiatric problems.

---

108 Ngim CH, Foo SC, Boey KW, Jeyaratnam J, Br J Med 49 (11): 782-790 (1992).

British Dental Journal

Fatal Mercury Intoxication in a Dental Surgery Assistant:

A 42-year-old dental surgery assistant with at least a 20-year history of exposure to mercury developed a rapidly fatal nephrotic syndrome. The high levels of mercury in the kidney, estimated by neutron activation analysis and demonstrated histologically, indicate that this was the result of mercury intoxication. Some unique features of the case are described and discussed. The warning is given that the risk of exposure to mercury in dental surgery is not trivial.[109]

CASRN

Neurobehavioral Effects

In talking about mercury...these neurobehavioral effects are memory, and visuomotor coordination speed. They are consistent with central and peripheral neurotoxicity and the TWA is considered consistent with central and peripheral neurotoxicity.[110]

Mercury Vapor Inhalation Inhibits Binding of GTP to Tubulin in Rat Brain: Similarity to a Molecular Lesion in Alzheimer Diseased Brain.

Neurotoxicology

Hg2+ interacts with brain tubulin and disassembles microtubules that maintain neurite structure. Since it is well known that Hg vapor (Hg^o) is continuously released from silver amalgam tooth fillings and is absorbed into brain, rats were exposed to Hg^o 4 h/day for 0,2,7, 14 and 28 d at 250 or 300 ug Hg/m3 air, concentrations present in mouth air

---

109 Cook TA, Yates PO, British Dental Journal 127:553:555 (1969).

110 Mercury, elemental CASRN 7439-97-6. (Chemical Abstracts Service Registry Number (CARSN). A unique number assigned to each molecule by the American Chemical Society.

of some humans with many amalgam fillings. Average rat brain Hg concentrations increased significantly (11-47 fold) with duration of Hg° exposure. By 14 d Hg° exposure, photoaffinity labeling of the B-subunit of the tubulin dimer with [a32P]8N3 GTP in brain homogenates was decreased 41-74 percent, upon analysis of SDS-PAGE autoradiograms. The identical neurochemical lesion of similar or greater magnitude is evident in Alzheimer brain homogenates from approximately 80 percent of patients, when compared to human age-matched neurological controls. Total tubulin protein levels remained relatively unchanged between Hg° exposed rat brains and controls, and between Alzheimer brains and controls. Since the rate of tubulin polymerization is dependent upon binding of GTP to tubulin dimers, we conclude that chronic inhalation of low-level Hg° can inhibit polymerization of brain tubulin essential for formation of microtubules.[111]

Journal of Neurochemistry 74(1): 231-6, 2000

What have rat brains got to do with humans?

The fact that mercury vapor (Hg°) dissembles the tubulin covering the synapses in rat brain is not satisfactory proof connecting mercury to Alzheimer's disease in humans.[112] Rats exposed to mercury display identical neurological changes in their brain tissue as observed in Alzheimer's. All mammals, e.g., a rat, elephant or the human brain, are structured in a similar manner.

---

111 James C. Pendergrass1, Boyd E. Haley1, Murray J. Vimy2, Stewart A. Winfield3 And Fritz L. Lorscheider 3,4 1College of Pharmacy, University of Kentucky, Lexington, KY, 40536; and Departments of 2Medicine and 3Medical Physiology, Faculty of Medicine, University of Calgary, Calgary, Alberta T2N 4N1, Canada. Neurotoxicology (18) (2) 315-324, 1997.

112 It is not legally possible to perform similar research on human beings because the subject would need to be euthanised.

Mercury Induces Cell Cytoxicity and Oxidative Stress and Increases B-Amyloid Secretion and Tau Phosphorylation in SHSY5Y Neuroblastoma Cells.

Concentrations of heavy metals, including mercury, have been shown to be altered in the brain and body fluids of Alzheimer's disease (AD) patients. To explore potential pathophysiological mechanisms we used an in vitro model system (SHSY5Y, neuroblastoma cells) and investigated the effects of inorganic mercury (HgC12) on oxidative stress, cell cytoxicity, B- amyloid production, and tau[113] phosphorylation.

We demonstrated that exposure of cells to 50 microgram/L (180 nM) HgCI2 for 30 min induces a 30 percent reduction in cellular glutathione (GSH) levels (n = 13, p < 0.001). Preincubation of cells for 30 min with 1 microM melatonin or premixing melatonin and HgCI2 appeared to protect cells from the mercury-induced GSH loss. Similarly, 3-(4,5- dimethylthiazo 1- 2-yl)- 2,5-diphenyltetrazolium bromide (MTT cytotoxicity assays revealed that 50 microgram/L HgCI2 for 24 h produced a 50 percent inhibition of MTT reduction (n = 9, p < 0.001). Again, melatonin preincubation protected cells from the deleterious effects of mercury, resulting in MTT reduction equaling control levels. The release of B- amyloid peptide (AB) 1-40 and 1-42 into cell culture supernatants after exposure to HgC12 was shown to be different: AB 1-40 showed maximal (15 .3ng/ml) release after 4 h, whereas AB 1-42 showed maximal (9.3 ng/ml) release after 6 h of exposure to mercury compared with untreated controls (n = 9, p < 0.001): Preincubation of cells with melatonin resulted in an attenuation of AB 1-40 and AB 1-42 release; -c:Tau phosphorylation was significantly increased in the presence of mercury (n=9, p <0.001), whereas melatonin preincubation reduced the phosphorylation to control values.

These results indicate that mercury may play a role in pathophysiological mechanisms of Alzheimer's disease.

---

113 Tau: subatomic particle similar to the electron

Dr. Boyd Haley, Professor and Chair of the Chemistry Department, at the University of Kentucky, Reports:

Glutamine synthetase is a definitive marker for Alzheimer's disease, whose function is to detoxify the brain by lowering its levels of glutamate and ammonia that are both toxic to the nervous system. Greatly elevated glutamine synthetase enzyme is present in the cerebral spinal fluid (CSF) of Alzheimer's patients. It is not found in the CSF of non-demented individuals who do not have Alzheimer's disease.

The glial cells that contain glutamine synthetase take up excess glutamate they convert to glutamine, which is non-toxic. Dr. William Markesberry, director of the Sanders Brown Center on Aging at the University of Kentucky Medical School, writes that mercury blocks the absorption of glutamate by the glial cells causing glutamate to rise, over-activating the neuronal cells and killing them.

Basic to all our findings is the following observation. Two very important brain nucleotide binding proteins, tubulin and creatine kinase (CK) show greatly diminished nucleotide binding ability and they are abnormally partitioned into the membrane fraction of brain tissue. What tubulin and CK have in common is that they both have a very reactive sulfthydryl, which, if modified, inhibits their biological activity. Mercury has a very high affinity for sulfthydryls and has been proven a potent inhibitor of both of these proteins' biological activity. Our laboratory demonstrated that tubulin had diminished biological activity in AD brain, and only AD brain etc.

Further research indicates that one can add various metals (Zn2+, Pb2+, Cu2+ etc.) to human brain homogenates to levels that do not affect nucleotide binding to tubulin. However, the addition of these metals lowers the concentration of Hg2+ that is required to totally abolish the nucleotide binding to tubulin. In other words, mercury is much more toxic in the presence of other metals that compete with mercury for binding sites on protective biomolecules (e.g., APO-E2 and E3, glutathione, metallothionine, etc.). If it cannot be directly proven that mercury causes Alzheimer's disease in humans, the combinations of other metals in the body potentialize the lethal effect of mercury causing Alzheimer's disease.

The Relationship of the Toxic Effects of Mercury to Exacerbation of the Medical Condition Classified as Alzheimer's disease. —Dr. Boyd Haley

Abstract: Mercury (II) or Hg2+ is neurotoxic and when exposed to normal brain tissue homogenates, is capable of causing many of the same biochemical aberrancies found in Alzheimer's diseased (AD) brain. Also, rats exposed to mercury vapor show some of these same aberrancies in their brain tissue. Specifically, the rapid inactivation of the brain thiol-sensitive enzymes tubulin, creatine kinase and glutamine synthetase occurs on the addition of low micromolar levels of Hg2+ or exposure to mercury vapor, and these same enzymes are significantly inhibited in AD brain. Further, extended Hg2+ exposure to neurons in culture has been shown to produce three of the widely accepted pathological diagnostic hallmarks of AD. These are elevated amyloid protein, hyper-phosphorylation of Tau, and formation of neurofibillary tangles. The hypothesis is that mercury and other blood-brain permeable toxicants that have enhanced specificity for thiol-sensitive enzymes are the etiological source of AD. Included in this category are other heavy metals such as lead and cadmium that act synergistically to enhance to toxicity of mercury and organic-mercury compounds, like thimerosal that is found in vaccines and other medicines. This hypothesis is also able to explain the genetic susceptibility to AD that is expressed through the APO-E gene family. Specifically, a reduction of APO-E gene types carrying cysteines decreases the ability to remove mercury and other thiol-reactive toxicants from the cerebrospinal fluid. This increases brain exposure to thiol-reactive toxicants and the risk of AD.

Neurobehavioral Effects From Exposure to Dental Amalgam Hg^o: New Distinction Between Recent Exposure and Hg Body Burden: FASEB

Potential toxicity from exposure to mercury vapor (Hg^o) from dental amalgam fillings is the subject of current public health debate in many countries. We evaluated potential central nervous system (CNS) toxicity associated with handling Hg-containing amalgam materials among dental personnel with very low-levels of Hg exposure (i.e., urinary Hg <4_g/1) applying a neurobehavioral test battery to evaluate CNS functions in relation to both recent exposure and Hg body burden. New distinctions between subtle preclinical effects on symptoms, mood, motor function and cognition were found associated with Hg body burden as compared with those associated with recent exposure. The pattern of results, comparable to findings previously reported among subjects with urinary Hg>50 _g/1, presents convincing new evidence of adverse behavioral effects associated with low Hg within range of that received by the general population.[114]

Neuroreport

Molecular Lesions Linked to Mercury

Inhalation of mercury vapor (Hg^o) inhibits binding of GTP to rat brain tubulin, thereby inhibiting tubulin polymerization into microtubules. A similar molecular lesion has also been observed in 80 percent of brains from patients with Alzheimer's disease (AD) compared to age-matched controls. However, the precise site and mode of action of Hg

---

114 Federation of American Societies for Experimental Biology (FASEB), 1998; 12:971-980. Diane Encheverria, HV Aposhian, JC Woods, NJ Heyer, MM Aposhian, AC Bittiner Jr., RK Mahurin, and M Cianciola; Batelle Centers for Public Health Research And Evaluation, Seattle; Dept. of Environmental Health, Univ. of WA, Seattle; Dept. of Molecular and Cellular Biology, Univ. of Arizona, Tucson; Dept. of Psychiatry, Univ. of WA, Seattle.

ions remain illusive. Therefore, the present study examined whether Hg ions could affect membrane dynamics of neurite growth cone morphology and behavior. Since tubulin is a highly conserved cytoskeletal protein in both vertebrates and invertebrates, we hypothesized that growth cones from animal species could be highly susceptible to Hg ions. To test this possibility, the identified, large Pedal A (PeA) neurons from the central ring ganglia of the snail Lymnaea stagnalis were cultured for 48 h in 2 ml brain conditioned medium (CM). Following neurite outgrowth, metal chloride solution (2 ml) of Hg, Al, Pb, Cd, or Mn (10-7 M) was pressure applied directly onto individual growth cones. Time-lapse images with inverted microscopy were acquired prior to, during, and after the metal ion exposure. We demonstrate that Hg ions markedly disrupted membrane structure and linear growth rates of imaged neurites in 77 percent of all nerve growth cones. When growth cones were stained with antibodies specific for both tubulin and actin, it was the tubulinmicrotubule structure that disintegrated following Hg exposure. Moreover, some denuded neurites were also observed to form neurofibrillary aggregates. In contrast, growth cone exposure to other metal ions did not affect growth cone morphology, nor was their motility rate compromised. To determine the growth suppressive effects of Hg ions on neuronal sprouting, cells were cultured either in the presence or absence of Hg ions. We found that in the presence of Hg ions, neuronal somata failed to sprout, whereas other metallic ions did not affect growth patterns of cultured PeA cells. We conclude that this visual evidence and previous biochemical data strongly implicate Hg as a potential etiological factor in neurodegeneration.[115]

Have links between mercury amalgam fillings and Alzheimer's been established?

If anyone still has any remaining doubts about this issue, see for your-

115 NeuroReport 12 (4) pg 733-737, March 2001, Christopher C. W. Leong, Naweed I. Syed, Fritz L. Lorscheider.

self. Go to http://movies.commons.ucalgary.ca/mercury. *How Mercury Causes Neurodegeneration* is a five-minute movie by the Canadian University of Calgary neuroscience team showing the myelin sheath disassembling, neurons dying and forming the neurofibillary tangles found in Alzheimer's disease in the presence of minute amounts of mercury.

Journal of the American College of Cardiology
Toxic Metals and Cardiomyopathy

Endomyocardial and thoracic-muscle concentrations of 32 trace elements were determined in biopsy samples from 13 patients with idiopathic dilated Cardiomyopathy (IDCM),[116] all without past or current exposure to trace elements, and in similar samples from 12 patients with valvular heart disease and 13 with iscehemic heart disease. Trace element concentrations were also determined in papillary and skeletal muscle from ten patients with mitral stenosis and normal left ventricular function and in left ventricular endomyocardial biopsies from four normal subjects. Compared with controls, all patients with IDCM had large increases in the concentrations of mercury (mean, 22,300-fold increase) and antimony[117] (mean, 12,840-fold increase) in myocardial but not in skeletal-muscle samples. The concentrations of other trace elements were elevated to a lesser degree in myocardial tissue (arsenic:[118] 250-fold increase; silver, gold, chromium, lanthanum and zinc: greater than 10-fold incrcases). Patients with secondary cardiac dysfunction had mild increases (5-fold or less) of myocardial trace elements and normal muscle concentrations.[119]

---

116 Cardiomyopathy: Disease of the myocardium: a primary disease of the heart muscle in the absence of known underlying cause.

117 A carcinogen.

118 A carcinogen.

119 Frustaci A, et al. Marked elevation of myocardial trace elements in idiopathic dilated Cardiomyopathy compared with secondary cardiac dysfunction. J Am Coll Cardiol 1999, 33:1575-1577.

Comment: This study showed that individuals with idiopathic dilated cardiomyopathy, but not those with secondary cardiac dysfunction, have enormous increases in the myocardial concentration of certain trace elements, particularly mercury, antimony and arsenic. Whether these increases are a cause or an effect of the disease is not known. However, increased concentrations of trace elements may adversely affect mitochondria activity and myocardial metabolism, resulting in clinical deterioration.

Smoking, mercury, other medical conditions and environmental toxins can cause arteriosclerosis within the arteries. Mercury is 22,000 times higher, postmortem, in the hearts of people who die from cardiomyopathy.

Journal of the American College of Cardiology

Marked Elevation of Myocardial Trace Elements in Idiopathic Dilated Cardiomyopathy Compared with Secondary Dysfunction

Objectives: We sought to investigate the possible pathogenic role of myocardial trace elements (TE) in patients with various forms of cardiac failure.

Background: Both myocardial TE accumulation and deficiency have been associated with the development of heart failure indistinguishable from an idiopathic dilated cardiomyopathy.

Methods: Myocardial and muscular content of 32 TE has been assessed in biopsy samples of 13 patients (pts) with clinical, hemodynamic and histologic diagnosis of idiopathic dilated cardiomyopathy (IDCM), all without past or current exposure to TE. One muscular and one left ventricular (LV) endomyocardial specimen from each patient, drawn with metal contamination-free technique, were analyzed by neutron activation analysis and compared with 1) similar surgical samples from patients with valvular (12 pts) and ischemic (13 pts) heart disease comparable for age and degree of LV dysfunction; 2) papillary and skeletal muscle surgical biopsies from 10 pts with mitral stenosis and normal LV function, and 3) LV endomyocardial biopsies from four normal subjects.

Results: A large increase (>10,000 times for mercury and antimony) of TE concentration has been observed in myocardial but not in muscular samples in all pts with IDCM. Patients with secondary cardiac dysfunction had mild increase (<5 times) of myocardial TE and normal muscular TE. In particular, in pts with IDCM mean mercury concentration was 22,000 times (178,400 ng/g vs. 8 ng/g), antimony 12,000 times (19,260 ng/g vs. 1.5 ng/g), gold 11 times (26 ng/g vs. 2.3 ng/g), chromium 13 times (2,300 ng/g vs. 177 ng/g) and cobalt 4 times (86.5 ng/g vs. 20 ng/g) higher than in control subjects.

Conclusions: A large, significant increase of myocardial TE is present in IDCM but not in secondary cardiac dysfunction. The increased concentration of TE in pts with IDCM may adversely affect mitochondrial activity and myocardial metabolism and worsen cellular function.[120]

(Author) After I took a homeopathic chelation remedy to drive mercury directly to the skin rather than allow mercury to go through the intestinal track and kidneys, within three weeks hundreds of shards of metal erupted slightly below my heart in a circle about the size of a coffee can lid. Might it be that the most cost-effective and least traumatic substitute for heart bypass surgery is a twelve-dollar homeo-

---

120 1Frustaci, A., 2Magnavita, N., 1Chimenti, C., 2Caldarulo, M., 3Sabbioni, E., 3Pietra, R., 4Cellini, C., 4Possati, G.F. and 1Maseri, A. 1Department of Cardiology, 2Department of Occupational Medicine, and 3Department of Cardiac Surgery, Catholic University, Rome Italy and CEC 4Environmental Institute Joint Research Center Ispra, Rome, Italy; Journal of the American College of Cardiology; Vol. 33, No. 6, 1999, pp. 1578-1583.

pathic remedy that drives mercury and other heavy metals directly to the skin? In Europe, some governments that provide National Health Insurance will not pay for heart bypass surgery until after the patient first tries chelation therapy.

Believe It or Not

From the ADA's Web Page.[121] April 1, 1998

Dental Amalgam: 150 years of Safety and Effectiveness

Used for more than 150 years,[122] dental amalgam (a.k.a. silver amalgam and mercury amalgam) is a safe, affordable and durable material used to restore the teeth of more than 100 million Americans. It contains a mixture of metals such as silver, copper and tin, in addition to mercury, which chemically binds these components into a hard, stable and safe substance.

Are dental amalgams safe?

Yes. Dental amalgam has been used in tooth restorations worldwide for more than 100 years. Studies have failed to find any link between amalgam restorations and any medical disorder. Amalgam continues to be a safe restorative material for dental patients.

Is it possible to have an allergic reaction to amalgam?

Only a very small number of people are allergic[123] to amalgam fill-

121 www.ada.org

122 This statement by the ADA is anecdotal evidence. Time lines are not proof of safety, e.g., tobacco is good for you because people have smoked since antiquity.

ings. Fewer than 100 cases have ever been reported. In these rare[124] instances, mercury may trigger an allergic response. Symptoms of amalgam allergy are very similar to a typical skin allergy.[125] The ADA further believes that specific treatment decisions involving dental patients are within the professional judgment of the individual practitioner. The Association does not require dentists to use dental amalgam, nor does it prohibit dentists from removing dental amalgam in appropriate cases. The Association does take the position that it is unethical for a dentist to remove serviceable dental amalgams from the non-allergic patient for the alleged purpose of removing toxic substances from the body, when such treatment is performed solely at the recommendation or suggestion of the dentist.

There exists no credible scientific evidence that dental amalgam, when used in restorations in the non-allergic patient, constitutes either a general health hazard or is in any way related to the cause or cure of any specific disease. Neither the Alzheimer's Association[126] nor the Multiple Sclerosis Society is aware of any scientific evidence that has shown a credible link between use of amalgam fillings and either disease.

Dr. William Tolhurst, the plaintiff in a case against the ADA involving

---

123 Use of word allergic is deliberately deceptive. The ADA uses the word allergic (implying allergy) instead of the accurate word poison, because allergy has a less "threatening" connotation to the public than poison. "It's a bizarre conversation we're having here. The ADA is trying to argue that a poison is not a poison." Dr. Alfred P. Zamm, Environmental Medicine.

124 See Chapter 4.

125 This ADA fairy tale boils down to President Harry Truman's euphemism, manure! I try to choose my words carefully and neither manure nor liar is adequate to describe the nonsense in this paragraph. See Chapter 4.

126 Edward Truschke, former executive director of the Alzheimer's Association, was very aware of the evidence linking mercury fillings to short-term memory loss.

placement of mercury fillings, became a quadriplegic after dental treatment. The legal finding of the court was:

In stating that the ADA "owes no legal duty of care to protect the public from allegedly dangerous products used by dentists," the Association was only articulating the legal principle that liability for negligence against a third party in a case like this is limited to those who guarantee the product at issue or help to market it. The Association does not fall into this category. Its only alleged involvement in the plaintiff's injury was providing information about amalgam to the dental profession.[127]

Designer Research

The University of Kentucky research by Saxe and Markesberry entitled "Alzheimer's disease, dental amalgam and mercury" and "Dental amalgam and cognitive function in older women: findings from the Nun Study" imply there is no connection between dental amalgam and Alzheimer's disease to justify the ADA's untenable position that mercury dental amalgam does not cause Alzheimer's disease.

Depending on how the research protocol is designed, how questions are posed and the integrity of the statistician, unscrupulous researchers can slant the outcome of the finished product to be anything the power structure desires. Two medical journals declined to publish either research paper. Obviously, there were real problems with the material because if the studies were genuine, the news would have made banner headlines in every major newspaper in the world. It appears the *Journal of the American Dental Association* published the two disingenuous research studies to confuse the public about mercury's connection to Alzheimer's disease.

---

127 Tolhurst v. Johnson and Johnson Consumer Products, Inc., et al.

Fifteen years ago, dentists said there was not sufficient evidence to justify discontinuing the use of mercury-amalgam fillings. Today there is solid scientific evidence confirming mercury-amalgam is a poison that causes neurodegeneration. It is up to the ADA to show us one genuine scientific study proving mercury is good for human tissue. "Don't tell us how long you've used mercury amalgam. Don't tell us how smart you are. Don't tell us how many credentials you have. Show us the science!"[128] "Where are your double-blind independent scientific studies that prove mercury, a known neurotoxic poison, causes no deleterious effect to human tissue[129] published in "genuine peer-reviewed medical journals" such as *FASEB*, Neuro Toxicology or Lancet? Neither the *New England Journal of Medicine* nor the *Journal of the American Dental Association* applies. The ADA journal is a trade publication. *The New England Journal of Medicine* has damaged its credibility.[130]

In order to make this message short enough for others to be willing to read, I have had to throw away a four-and-one-half to five-foot stack of research papers from all over the world about mercury's poisonous properties. The computer database of Professor Hanson[131] contains over 14,000 research papers about mercury toxicity from mercury-amalgam dental fillings. Cornell University's database by itself contains 3,138 research papers and MSDS sheets about mercury toxicity. The fact that the ADA has stonewalled this issue is outrageous. The ADA's lies and cover-up have caused dentists to poison more than 80 percent of our population. If anyone other than a dentist put mercury in a person's mouth, the perpetrator would be charged with assault.

---

128 Jim Love, attorney.

129 John Moore: Former Boeing engineer who was poisoned by mercury dental fillings.

130 Nearly half of the drug reviews published in the NEJM since 1997 had undisclosed financial support from companies marketing the drugs.

131 Department of Zoophysiology, University of Lund Helgonvagen 3B S-233 62 Lund, Sweden.

The Parallax View

Let's take this scenario up several levels. Suppose that you were a foreign intelligence officer looking for a perfect undetectable poison to destroy an enemy in a way that brought no repercussions to you. Suppose that your research scientists discovered a neurotoxic substance that is one of the most lethal non-radioactive elements in the Periodic Table and that it has an affinity for brain and neurological tissue.

The onset of clinical symptoms from chronic low-level mercury poisoning are so vague and insidious that physicians are unable to detect the cause of the patient's distress. One person may develop schizophrenia, another tremors (Parkinson's), another Alzheimer's, multiple sclerosis or cancer because the poison heads for the weakest organ and weakest gene.

If you could induce your enemy's dentists to insert this diabolical toxin into their patient's oral cavity two inches from the brain in eighty-five percent of your enemy's population, you would wreak havoc on the whole fabric of their society. You could put hundreds of thousands of their citizenry in mental hospitals. You could destroy entire families. Sick people are inefficient, troublesome workers. They fill the welfare rolls. They fill the prisons. You could cause hundreds of millions of dollars to be spent supporting institutionalized mental patients and imprisoned no-accounts. You would force the enemy to spend billions of dollars on unnecessary pharmaceuticals and medical bills before poisoned patients expire. In addition, sick under-employed workers cannot pay taxes. The best part is that the last person anyone would suspect of poisoning them is their dentist.

If the above parody were true, if it was discovered that any foreign nation caused millions of our population the devastation I just described, we would declare war. This discovery would be considered "A Day In Infamy." Unfortunately, the only incongruity in this whole story is there is no foreign intelligence officer involved. I wish there were. It would make the following information more palatable.

This is what has been covered up:

1. The primary cause of Alzheimer's is iatrogenic disease, dentist-induced disease, from mercury amalgam dental fillings that poison the brain and central nervous system. Methyl mercury vapor has an affinity for brain and neurological tissue and easily passes through the blood brain barrier.

2. Degenerative diseases caused by root-canal infection have been covered up or ignored for 80 years.

3. Alzheimer's is not incurable. If an Alzheimer's sufferer can carry on a halfway reasonable conversation for five minutes, Alzheimer's is reversible.[132] Every once in a while someone tugs on my sleeve in a store, a restaurant or after a speaking engagement and tells me that I have saved his or her life.

The most accurate name for Alzheimer's disease should be "Chronic Low-level Mercurial Poisoning." Mercury poisoning from mercury amalgam dental fillings is a causative factor in the majority of people diagnosed with schizophrenia, Alzheimer's and neurological disease. Mercury overwhelms the immune system allowing infectious micro-organisms in cavitations and root canals to cause many other devastating diseases.[133]

Those of us who have had our lives turned upside down by mercury poisoning could live with the fact that our dentists made an appalling mistake in not recognizing the toxicity of mercury sooner. What we will not tolerate is that once the ADA recognized there were problems with amalgam, they did everything within their power to stonewall the fact that mercury fillings were poisoning dental patients. At the

132 I couldn't carry on a halfway normal conversation for two minutes. At times, the longest I could hold on to a string of thought was less than 30 seconds.

133 Read Chapter 2 and appendix XIII.

very least, dentists should have warned dental patients of the toxicity of mercury and its danger to the brain and central nervous system.

Recent legislation by the state of Maine orders dentists to inform patients about the presence of mercury in dental amalgam. See Appendix VIII for the press release. Twenty-five States, including Washington and Oregon, are introducing bills that will force dentists to reveal the known side effects of mercury in mercury dental fillings. California has already passed similar legislation.

Where has the FDA been in all this? They know everything within this book. The amalgam issue is another "Libby Asbestos Mine Disaster" swept under the rug. True or not, to a broad spectrum of the American population, it appears campaign financing and public relation firms have compromised the government agencies that are supposed to protect the public interest. The question that begs an answer is: Why has the FDA been sitting on its hands? Who shut the FDA up?

The Material Safety Data Sheets (MSDS) by dental amalgam manufacturers and United States government agencies such as the FDA, EPA and ATSDR have been revised to the point that they have become almost meaningless in 2000 and 2001. The FDA went so far as to publish a disingenuous white paper telling the public there is no creditable scientific evidence that mercury fillings hurt anyone that mimics the doublespeak in George Orwell's *1984*. Could the unprecedented advocacy be because the FDA colluded with the ADA to grandfather silver fillings without the scientific proof of safety and efficacy any other drug put into the human body has to prove prior to distribution? Or, is it because the FDA has set the government up for more potential economic liability than all the money that exists in the United States? The mercury amalgam issue is a political hydrogen bomb, because once the general public realizes mercury amalgam dental fillings have killed more people, both military and civilian, than all the wars in the 20th Century, politicians who had their hands in the dental industry's pockets might as well retire—they will never be re-elected.

Apparently the good old boys realized that if the straight talk in the former Internet web page MSDS sheets about mercury amalgam was available to the general public, it might force manufacturers to discontinue using mercury in approximately 4,000 products from light switches, mercury-impregnated plastic and leather used in automobile interiors to amalgam dental fillings.

How was it possible to circumnavigate the mercury amalgam issue?

The FDA did that by separating mercury from the other metals used in dental fillings, because the dentist does not mix mercury into amalgam until just before it is placed into the oral cavity. Any high school science student knows mercury is the deadliest non-radioactive poison in the Periodic Table. That's why dentists refer to amalgam as silver amalgam instead of mercury amalgam, its proper name.[134] In addition, because of the FDA's chicanery, the ADA is not even forced to supply a manufacturers package insert to inform their dental patients about the side effects of chronic low-level mercurial poisoning causing the dental patient to be unable to recognize the contra-indications of mercury in time to protect their health.

One hundred and seventy years ago, the average dentist was a wood carver, jewelry engraver, barber or mortician. Anyone could apprentice under a journeyman dentist who probably knew less about the toxicity of the materials they used in their practice than journeymen tuck-pointers know about the materials they use to repair leaky masonry buildings today. For example, any construction worker with a computer can read MSDS sheets about toxic chemicals they are exposed to on the job and the safety of materials they install in new buildings.

---

134 The proper scientific name for any amalgam compound is its highest metal content.

Autopsy studies conducted by the Swedish Karolinska Institute and the University of Southern California Dental School indicate people who had seven mercury amalgam dental fillings, the number in the mouth of the average American, postmortem,[135] had four times more mercury in their brain tissue and nine times more mercury in their kidneys than people who did not have mercury amalgam fillings. At one time I had 28.

Why would any sane person put toxic waste in his or her mouth? More importantly, why would parents allow a dentist to poison their children? The answer is—they didn't know.

Informed Consent

Every pharmaceutical medication distributed in the United States has a package insert to inform doctors, pharmacists and patients of the known side effects to their medications and to answer any questions the patient might ask. To obtain a package insert, all anyone needs to do is ask the pharmacist for a copy. This is precisely the type of information dentists should have provided dental patients before they placed mercury amalgam in anyone's mouth. Instead, the ADA colluded with the FDA to cover up mercury's poisonous properties. State dental boards and dental societies have done their utmost to suppress Informed Consent and continually harass and revoke licenses of dentists who advise their patients about the toxicity of mercury amalgam fillings. The Washington State Dental Board is presently trying to suppress the cavitation issue.[136] In California, the American Civil Liberties Union (ACLU) is in the process of joining this fray under the First Amendment right to free speech.

---

135 The Journal of the American Dental Association, Volume 129, Page 1471, October 1998.

136 The average American citizen has 12 mercury amalgam fillings. From the above research, it appears by the time people die they have lost five teeth that contained mercury amalgam fillings.

Oregon Dental Board Rescinds Gag Rule 3/8/2002

Today the Oregon Dental Board voted unanimously to rescind a rule that has been on their books since 1990 that effectively gagged dentists from discussing the potentially harmful effects of mercury exposure emanating from mercury-amalgam dental fillings. The issue was brought to a head by the ACLU protesting to the State Attorney General that the dental board's rule was a clear violation of a dentist's right to free speech under the U.S. and Oregon constitutions.

Orwellian Doublespeak: Informed Consent and the Law - JADA [137]

"It is a well-recognized principle of law that every adult of sound mind has a right to determine what will be done with his or her own body. From this principle, the concept that a patient may not be treated without his or her informed consent is usually considered a form of negligence. Failure of the dentist to disclose the risks of treatment can be the basis of the patient's malpractice claim."

Dentists are put in an untenable position: if they inform their patients that mercury is a noxious poison that does not belong in anyone's mouth, the ADA, in collusion with state dental boards, will work to have their licenses to practice dentistry revoked. If the patient's health is damaged, it is the dentists whom the ADA plans to let hang out to dry in the wind all by themselves. Ask any ADA dentist if mercury fillings are poisonous. They will do the politician's slide-step, side-step. Tell the dentist all you want is a simple yes or no answer: Is mercury poisonous?

---

137 The Journal of the American Dental Association, Volume 129, Page 1471, October 1998

It is the dentist who will be impacted by the consequences.

In a newspaper article entitled "Brush with Danger" in the San Francisco East Bay Monthly, June 1997, Mark Anderson reported, "The scientific and medical evidence available suggests that the mercury amalgam issue is an internal Love Canal waiting to be exposed. The San Francisco Bar Association indicated that if a definitive link could be found between Alzheimer's, Amyotrophic lateral sclerosis (ALS), multiple sclerosis or Parkinson's, the legal implications would be staggering."

Who Will Wind up Paying the Bill?

There is going to be a bill, you know. Dentists expect the deep pockets of their insurance companies to protect them. Normally I would agree, except that in 1987 the ADA made it unethical for a dentist to remove mercury amalgam fillings from the patient for the alleged purpose of removing toxic substances (mercury) from the body. They pressured dental boards to revoke the licenses of dentists who were outspoken critics of mercury-dental amalgam. That is proof of cover-up any jury can understand. The bottom line is that the ADA has committed fraud. Unless collusion can be proved between their insurance companies and the ADA, the insurance industry will be off the hook.

Neurobehavioral effects from exposure to dental amalgam Hg^o: new distinctions between recent exposure and Hg body burden

Diana Echeverria, H., Vasken Aposhian, James S. Woods, Nicholas J. Heyer, Mary M. Aposhian, Alvah Bittner JR, Roderick K. Mahurin, and Margaret Cianciola.

Battelle Centers for Public Health Research and Evaluation, Seattle,

Washington 98105.

Department of Environmental Health, University of Washington, Seattle, Washington 98195 Department of Molecular and Cellular Biology, University of Arizona, Tucson, Arizona 85721.

Department of Psychiatry, University of Washington, Seattle, Washington 98195.

Potential toxicity from exposure to mercury vapor (Hg^o) from dental amalgam fillings is the subject of current public health debate in many countries. We evaluated potential central nervous system (CNS) toxicity associated with handling Hg-containing amalgam materials among dental personnel with very low levels of Hg^o exposure (i.e., urinary Hg <4 μg/l), applying a neurobehavioral test battery to evaluate CNS functions in relation to both recent exposure and Hg body burden. New distinctions between subtle preclinical effects on symptoms, mood, motor function, and cognition were found associated with Hg body burden as compared with those associated with recent exposure. The pattern of results, comparable to findings previously reported among subjects with urinary Hg >50 μg/l, presents convincing new evidence of adverse behavioral effects associated with low Hg^o exposures within the range of that received by the general population.

DENTISTS BE WARNED

April 30, 2002

By KOMO Staff & News Services

Mercury Fillings May Be Affecting Dentists

Tue Apr 30, 10:33 AM ET

LONDON (Reuters) - Dentists are more likely to suffer memory and kidney problems which could be due to long-term exposure to mercury in tooth fillings, doctors said on Tuesday.

A study of 180 dentists by researchers at the Glasgow Royal Infirmary in Scotland found the dentists had up to four times the normal level of mercury in their urine and nails and had more kidney disorders and memory lapses than the general public.

"We found several differences in the health and cognitive functioning between our dentists and the control group," Dr. Ewan Macdonald said in a report in the *Journal of Occupational and Environmental Medicine.*

"These differences could not be directly attributed to their exposure to mercury, but as mercury exposure at higher levels is known to cause similar health effects an association cannot be ruled out," he added.

Mercury has been used in dentistry for about 150 years but some dentists and esearchers believe the fillings can give off harmful vapors that can be dangerous for dentists and patients.

Critics of the fillings claim the mercury can poison the body and lead to health problems affecting the kidneys and other organs and neurological diseases such as Alzheimer's.

But dental associations say it is safe when mixed with other metals and there are no scientific studies to prove a link between the filling and health problems.

The researchers in Glasgow compared mercury levels in urine, hair and nail samples and the results of psychomotor skills, response times, word recall and health problems of the 180 dentists and an equal number of volunteers.

The dentists had higher levels of the metal in their bodies, reported more health problems and did worse on the tests than the volunteers.

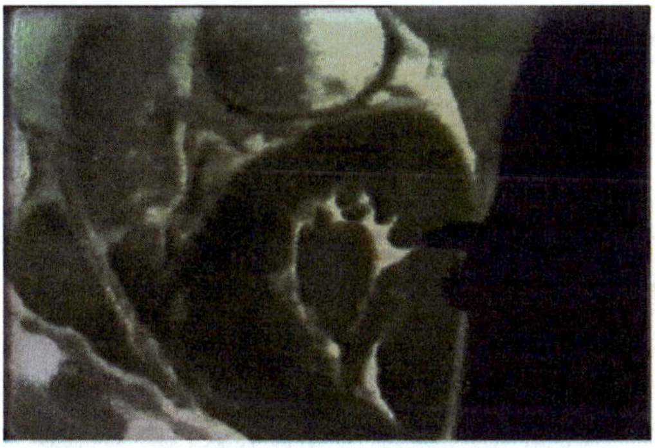

The black area of the monkey's heart that the doctor is pointing to is contaminated with mercury.

Page 2636 of the 1999 17th edition of the Merck Manual connects mercury poisoning to renal (kidney) failure and perforation of the intestinal wall. One of the MSDS sheets at the beginning of this chapter plainly states mercury poisoning causes renal failure. Mercury settles in the heart, brain tissues, the groin area and reproductive organs, ankles, fat and connective tissues. It poisons every cell in the body.

I had Alzheimer's disease. Several months ago two doctors informed me that I have nephropathy, a supposedly fatal form of kidney disease. One of my former dentists has the beginning symptoms of Parkinson's disease.

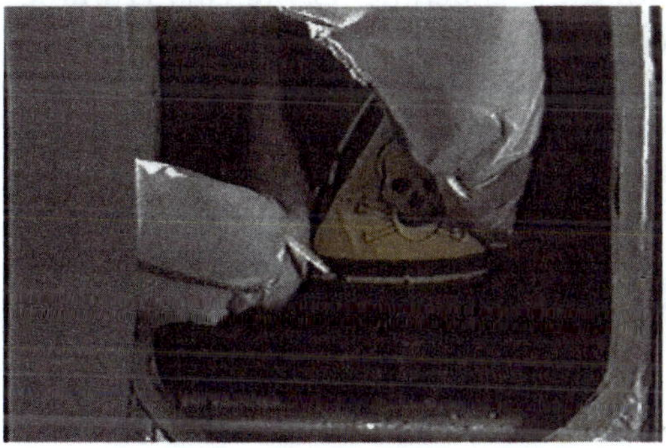

The universal sign for death

No rational person who truly understands the poisonous nature of mercury would willingly choose to have mercury placed in his or her teeth or any other part of their body. Anyone who advocates putting mercury in the body is either irrational or does not understand the poisonous nature of mercury. It is not a matter of—if mercury is safe, it's that mercury is poisonous."

– Dr. Genung

The World Health Organization reviewed all of the research and could not find any level of mercury that did not cause cellular effects.

— Dr. Murray Vimy

Let's Keep It Simple

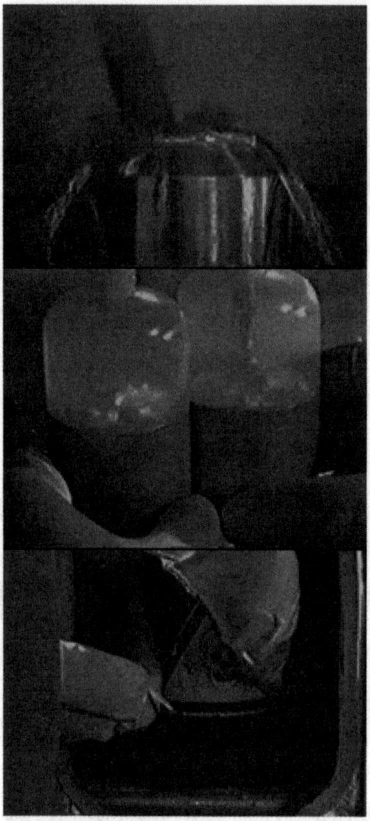

"If you have something that's been put in your mouth that you can't dispose of in a waste basket without breaking environmental protection laws, there's no point in keeping it around, there's no point in taking that type of risk-there's no point in exposing people to any level of mercury toxicity if you don't have to.

"There is no doubt in my mind that low-levels of mercury present in the brain causes neuronal cell death, and this could lead to dementia which would be similar to Alzheimer's disease. We can't go inside a living human being and look at their brain, so we have to work outside, and do scientific experiments such as we've done. And to the best that we can determine with these experiments, mercury is a time bomb in the brain, waiting to have an effect. If it's not bothering someone when they're young, especially when they age it can turn into something quite disastrous."

— Dr. Boyd Haley

Common Complaints of Mercury Toxicity

Dr. Hal Huggins generated the following list of symptoms from dental patients he treated for mercury toxicity. For further information, Dr. Huggins' Web page is http://www.hugnet.com.

Percentage of 1320 Respondents Indicating Presence of Symptoms

Symptoms	Percentage
Unexplained irritability	73.3*
Constant or very frequent periods of depression	72.0*
Numbness and tingling in the extremities	67.3**
Frequent urination during the night	64.5**
Unexplained chronic fatigue	63.1*
Cold hands and feet, even in moderate/warm weather	62.6***
Bloated feeling most of the time	60.6
Difficulty remembering or use of memory	58.0**
Sudden, unexplained or unsolicited anger	55.5*
Constipation on a regular basis	54.6
Difficulty in making simple decisions	54.2*

Tremors or shakes of hands, feet, head, etc.	52.3*
Twitching of the face and other muscles	52.3**
Frequent leg cramps	49.1***
Constant or frequent ringing or noise in the ears	47.8**
Becoming out of breath easily	43.1
Frequent or reoccurring heartburn	42.5**
Excessive itching	40.8*
Unexplained rashes, skin irritation	40.4*
Constant or frequent metallic taste in mouth	38.7*
Being jumpy, jittery, nervous	38.1*
Constant death wish or suicidal intent	37.3
Frequent insomnia	36.4**
Unexplained chest pains	35.6*
Tachycardia	32.4
Unexplained fluid retention	28.2*
Burning sensation on tongue	20.8*
Having headaches just after eating	20.1*
Frequent diarrhea	14.9

Author's comments:

* *At one time or another I have experienced these symptoms*

** *I still have these problems*

*** *These symptoms are severe*

Parke-Davis List of Symptoms

The Parke-Davis Continuing Pharmacy Education Course lists the early warning signs of Alzheimer's disease in the following manner:

Cognitive	Behavioral
Memory loss affecting job or household skills	Suspiciousness, Paranoia
Time/place disorientation	Increased appetite
Language problems	Loss of initiative
Difficulty with abstract thinking	Agitation
Poor judgment	Personality changes
Misplacing things	Liability of mood
Depression	(rapidly changing)

Compare Parke-Davis symptoms with the above symptoms of chronic low-level mercurial poisoning.

My List of Symptoms

This list is generated by the author and is found on the Internet at http://www.beatingchronicdisease.com.

Mercury poisoning and toxic chemicals cause Alzheimer's sufferers many common medical and mental problems. Following is a list of some of the symptoms routinely seen in these patients:

Irritability and inexplicable explosive behavior

Endogenous depression

Emotional instability

Low, or no stomach acid

Candida overgrowth

H-pylori (Helicobacter pylori)

Excessive belching and flatulence

Putrefaction, parasites, flukes, fungus, etc.

Malnutrition

Tiredness and chronic fatigue

Leaky-gut syndrome

Food allergies and chemical sensitivities

Poisoning of the liver

Dry flaky skin

Abnormal white cell blood count ranging from 10,000 to 22,000 mm

Discoloration of the genital organs

The subclinical signs of mercury poisoning are: short-term memory problems, white spots on the fingernails, hangnails, inability to remember dreams, cracks or holes on the tongue, and frequent urination.

There are other subclinical signs of mercury poisoning, but these are the complaints that I most often hear from persons seeking information about short-term memory loss.

What are Nutritional Supplements?

Vitamins are minute amounts of organic substances the human body cannot live without that are found in natural foodstuffs, or sometimes produced synthetically. For example, Vitamin A prevents night blindness. Correction of sugar, fat and protein excesses and controlled supplementation with pyridoxine (Vitamin B6), magnesium, chromium and coenzyme Q10 prevent diabetes and arteriosclerosis.[138] Vitamins B1, B3,[139] B6, pantothenic acid, Vitamin C, Vitamin E and Vitamin B12 are used to treat schizophrenia.[140] Dr. Abram Hoffer tells a story about Canadian prisoners of war who were starved during WW II who developed schizophrenia. He treated the former soldiers with megadoses of the above vitamins. Schizophrenia went into remission until they discontinued their regimen of vitamin supplementation but recovered after they resumed their course of therapy.

138 Dr. John T.A, Ely, "Unrecognized Pandemic Subclinical Diabetes of the Affluent Nations: Causes, Cost and Prevention," *Journal of Orthomolecular Medicine, Second Quarter 1966-Vol-11, Number 2.*

139 Orthomolecular physicians are beginning to suspect the B3 dose Dr. Hoffer recommends (1,000 mg after each meal at older ages) might be excessive. Try taking 200 mg after each meal for a while. There is a level above which every substance becomes toxic-even water.

140 Dr. Abram Hoffer, Dr. Morton Walker, *Smart Nutrients*, Avery, New York, 1994.

Malnutrition

If you have brain allergies, you also have acute malnutrition. Your digestive system does not function properly and your brain is starving.[141] That is one of the reasons the Alzheimer's brain loses 20 to 30 percent of its former weight before the patient expires. Another reason the Alzheimer's patient is deficient in vitamins and minerals is because mercury toxicity and diabetes cause Alzheimer's patients to urinate more often than normal, depleting the nutritional supplements they do ingest. All mercury toxic sufferers have low stomach acid. Antacids are not the solution. They temporarily relieve distress all right, but complicate the problem by causing the patient to believe indigestion is caused by excessive stomach acid when in fact, it is caused by low, and in some cases, no stomach acid. If Alzheimer's sufferers do not straightaway deliver enough of the right nutritional supplements to the brain, they will become too incapacitated to take the necessary steps to reverse the disease process and heal themselves.

Along this same line, diabetes is known to cause sudden blindness. My eyesight was rapidly failing and I was going blind. My blood glucose levels have averaged less than 102 for months and my eye doctor did not have the slightest clue as to the cause of my distress. I have known for years that my stomach acid is more neutral than water and suspected malnutrition might be the origin of the symptoms I was experiencing, so I went to a health food store and ordered several small carrots, cabbage, broccoli and one clove of garlic to be juiced. The following morning when I awoke, my eyesight had dramatically improved. As long as I stick with vegetable juices that are low in sugar content, my eyesight remains normal. Read *Make Your Juicer*

---

141 In the case of schizophrenia, have the internist check the thickness of the patient's blood. I had a client who was hospitalized five years before a smart psychiatrist realized the cause of his distress was because his blood was too thick. The fellow was released within one week. Very likely, atherosclerosis was also involved. Garlic is an excellent blood thinner. I mix one clove of garlic in my vegetable juice every other day. Is the patient drinking enough water?

Your Drug Store by Dr. Laura Newman, Benedict Lust Publications, New York, NY, 10156. Probably the best nutritional study ever conducted was by Dr. Francis Pottenger Jr., Pottenger's Cats: A Study in Nutrition, available from the Price-Pottenger Nutrition Foundation, P.O. Box 2614, La Mesa, CA 92004. If you are not thinking clearly, buy the video.

The AMA recommends all adults take daily vitamin supplements, reversing their 20-year anti-vitamin policy because they discovered we are not receiving enough vitamins from our diets.[142]

I wonder why they said, "adults?" What about our children?

A couple of weeks ago, I ran out of the vitamin B complex I have taken for years and temporarily substituted what is touted as being a high-quality synthetic B complex vitamin whose manufacturer covers a large percentage of the shelf space. I forgot to use the kinesiology test and find even if I take three times the amount of my regular product, my tongue still cracks—which, at least for me, is a definite sign of malabsorption.

A fellow suffering short-term memory loss, who couldn't even tell a club from a spade, took many of the same vitamins and minerals I do for less than three weeks, is now able to beat his wife at bridge again. A daughter of a 93-year-old woman wrote that her mother regained her short-term memory after reading *Beating Alzheimer's* by taking nutritional supplements.

One of the most difficult problems I had was putting together the right combination of vitamins and minerals to regenerate my immune system and shoo away muddled thinking.

The most accurate thing I can tell readers about nutritional supplements is to seek the most qualified orthomolecular psychiatrist or physician they can find and follow his or her advice.

---

142 JAMA, 2002; NO. 23, VOL. 287.

For those who want to know, some of the vitamins and minerals that I take are:

Digestive Enzymes-every time I put food in my mouth

Essential Botanicals

Cellular-DX

Choleste-care

Essential Minerals

OPC

Uña de gato

Thiamin (B-1)

Niacin (B-3)

Pyridoxin (B-6)

Pantothenic Acid

Vitamin C

Vitamin E

Beta Carotene

Alpha Lipoic Acid[143]

---

143 Alpha Lipoic Acid is an important antioxidant and chelating agent, which will be discussed in Appendix IV.

What is MSM?

By Dr. Stanley Jacobs[144]

MSM (methylsulfonylmethane, also known as dimethylsulfone) is a naturally occurring nutrient, a sulfur compound found in normal human diets and those of virtually all other vertebrates. In its purified form it is an odorless, essentially tasteless, white, water-soluble, crystalline solid. Its chemical formula is (CH3) 2SO2.

Where Is MSM Found?

It has been suggested by one of the world's most prominent atmospheric chemists that MSM and its related compounds, DMSO (dimethylsulfoxide) and DMS (dimethylsulfide), provide the source for 85 percent of the sulfur found in all living organisms. The cycle of these naturally occurring sulfur compounds begins in the ocean where microscopic plants and animals called plankton release sulfur compounds called dimethylsulfonium salts. These salts are transformed in the ocean water into the very volatile compound dimethylsulfide (DMS), which escapes from the ocean water as a gas and rises into the upper atmosphere. Here, in the presence of ozone and high-energy ultraviolet light, the DMS is converted into its cousins DMSO and MSM. Unlike the DMS, both DMSO and MSM are very soluble in water, and they return to the surface of the earth in the rain. Plants take up the two compounds very rapidly into their root systems, concentrating them up to one hundred fold. MSM itself and the sulfur it

144 Oregon Health Sciences, Portland, Oregon. Reprinted with permission of author.

contains are incorporated into the plant structure. Through the process of plant metabolism, the MSM, along with the other sulfur compounds it has spawned, are ultimately mineralized and transported back to the sea, and the sulfur cycle begins again.

MSM has been found in the blood and adrenal glands of cows. Cow's milk contains between two and six parts per million MSM. It has been found in green vegetables.

Why Is MSM Important For Us?

MSM is found naturally in the human body. It occurs in the blood and in the other organs as well. It has been detected in normal human urine. The natural level of MSM in the circulatory system of the adult human male is about 0.2 parts per million. Normal human adults excrete from four to 11 mg MSM per day in their urine. In mammals, the concentration of MSM in the body's various storehouses decreases with age, possibly as a result of changing diet and metabolism. Some research suggests that there is a minimum concentration of MSM that must be maintained in the body to preserve the normal function and structure.

The MSM we ingest in fresh fruits, vegetables and milk contributes essential sulfur for synthesis of connective tissue, enzymes and immunoglobulin. Sulfur is an important element in formation and good health of hair and nails.

How Does The Body Utilize MSM?

Experiments using MSM that contains radiolabeled sulfur (35/S) have shown that after ingestion, MSM gives up its sulfur to form the collagen and keratin of the hair and nails, to form the essential amino acids methionine, cysteine, and to form the serum proteins.

What About Toxicity?

MSM is rated as one of the least toxic substances in biology, similar in toxicity to water. Common table salt is much more toxic than MSM. The lethal dose (LD50) of MSM for mice is over 20g/kg of body weight. When MSM was administered orally to human volunteers, no toxic effects were observed at the intake levels up to one gm/kg of weight per day for 30 days (10). Intravenous injections of 0.5 gm/kg daily for five days a week, three to six days, produced no measurable toxicity in human subjects. MSM has been widely tested as a food ingredient without any reports of allergic reactions. An unpublished Oregon Health Sciences University study of the long-term toxicity of MSM over a period of six months showed no toxic effects. More than 12,000 patients have been treated at the Oregon Health Sciences University with MSM at levels above two grams daily with no serious toxicity (10).

How Does The Body Get Its MSM?

MSM is a natural component of many fresh fruits, vegetables, seafood and meat. It is also found in tea, coffee and chocolate. Cow's milk is a particularly rich source of MSM. However, heat and processing can reduce the MSM in foods.

What Can MSM Do For Us?

Scientists don't yet know precisely the normal functions of MSM in the human body. At the Oregon Health Sciences University there have been many observations of what it can achieve in the way of health and well-being when taken as a dietary supplement in doses of 250 to 750 milligrams per day. The following are some conditions helped by MSM.

Response to allergies: Oral MSM has alleviated the allergic response to pollen and to foods. The anti-allergic property of MSM is on par with or better than the traditional antihistaminic preparations.

Control of hyperacidity: Patients who have used antacids and histamine receptor antagonists to control hyperacidity can employ MSM with excellent results.

Control of constipation: Patients with chronic constipation have prompt and continuing relief with a daily supplement of 100 to 500 mg per day orally.

Some Clinical and Laboratory Studies on MSM

There have been many studies conducted under controlled conditions that show some of the potential that MSM has as a therapeutic agent. These include studies on snoring, lupus, breast cancer and rheumatoid arthritis.

Lovelock, J.E. et al., Nature, Vol. 237, 452, 1972

Ruzicka, L. et al., Helv chim acte, Vol 23, 550, 1940

Pfiffner, J.J. and North, H.G., J. Bill Chem, Vol 131, 731, 1940

Williams, K.I.H. et al., Proc Soc Exp Biol & Med, Vol.122, 865, 1966

Pearson T.W. et al., Agnic Food Chem, Vol. 29, 1089, 1981

Williams, K.I.H. et al., Arch Biochem Biophys, Vol. 113, 251, 1966

Jacob, S.W. and Hershler, R., Ann N.Y. Acad Sci, Vol. 411. XIII, 1983

Richmond, V.L., J Nutrition, Vol. 116, No. 6, June 1986

Deichman, W.B. & Gerarde, H.W., editors, Toxicology of Drugs and Chemicals, 4th Edition. Academic Press 1969

Jacobs, S.W., Oregon Health Science University, Portland, Oregon, Personal Communication

Bennett, J.C. & Plum, F., editors, Cecil Textbook of Medicine. 20th Edition, W.B. Saunders Co., 1996

Siegel, J.M., Oregon Health Sciences University, Portland, Oregon, Personal communication

McCabe, D. et al., Arch Surg. Vol. 121, 1455, 1986

O'Dwyer, P.J. et al., Cancer, Vol. 62, 944, 1988

Morton, J.I. & Moore, R.D., Federation of American Societies for Experimental Biology, 69th Annual Meeting, April 21-26, 1985, 692, 198

Baths

Simple Clay Bath

By Lauana Lei[145]

A few years ago I was diagnosed with heavy metal and chemical poisoning. Among the many toxic substances in my body, mercury from fillings in my teeth was a major culprit.

It was recommended that I have all my fillings replaced (a major undertaking)!

After undergoing live cell/dry cell analysis, I was told I needed twenty chelation treatments (a drip-intravenous therapy) at $100 per session (much more expensive today), which meant an additional $2,000. To confirm the diagnosis, I had a frozen sample of my blood sent to a special laboratory in Colorado. The lab analysis showed an alarming variety of poisons in my body including dioxin, mercury, aluminum, cadmium, arsenic, lead, chlorine and copper. On a scale of 1 to 10 (ten being the most toxic) seven elements registered 7 or more. Where, you might ask, did all those metals come from?

Dioxin, one of the deadliest substances known, is sprayed on coffee and vegetable fields in Costa Rica where I had visited for several months. Dioxin is also found in many lawn fertilizers.

Mercury, besides leaking from tooth fillings, is also found in fish, cos-

145 Copyright 2000, USA, reprinted with permission

metics, soil, pesticides, film (photos and negatives), paint and plastics.

Aluminum is used in soft drink cans, cookware, cheeses, white flour, baking powder and deodorants.

Cadmium is contained in cigarette smoke, gasoline, steel cooking pans and metal pipes.

Arsenic may be present in some types of rice, salt and smog (industrial pollution).

Lead is found in dyes, gasoline, paint, plumbing, pottery, insecticides, tobacco smoke, textiles and scrap metal.

Carbon Monoxide of course comes from auto exhaust, cigarette smoke and smog.

A number of these substances may also be found in our water. All of us are exposed to countless chemicals and metals every day of our lives.

There are over 70,000 chemicals being used in commercial production in the U.S. Sixty-five thousand of them are classified by the Environmental Protection Agency as potentially or definitely hazardous to human health, according to Dr. Steven Schechter, author of *Fighting Radiation and Chemical Pollutants With Foods, Herbs and Vitamins:* Documented Natural Remedies That Boost Your Immunity and Detoxify. He noted new chemicals are being tested in the U.S. at the rate of 6,000 per week.

In the words of medical researcher Dr. Alan Levine, the vast increase of chemicals in our environment, foods and medicines has greatly altered our body's ability to rid itself of toxins.

The Search for Alternatives

Having neither health insurance nor the money to pay these expensive treatments, I began to search for alternative ways to eliminate these poisons (a major cause of immune system breakdown) and thus, a source of various diseases.

I learned that certain toxic elements could be removed by taking specific combinations of minerals and vitamins. For example, a daily regimen of six magnesium oxide[146] tablets plus a teaspoon of calcium/magnesium powder taken with fresh lemon juice was said to rid the body of arsenic (eventually). But at this rate, it could take years to clear all the chemicals and metals from my body.

My search led me to a book, *Using Energy to Heal*, by Windell Hoffman. Through his own research, Hoffman found that a special bentonite (a very fine volcanic clay) used in a bath could actually draw out toxic chemicals through the pores of the skin. After many experiments he concluded that optimum results are obtained by immersing oneself in a tub of very warm water mixed with special bentonite clay for exactly 20 minutes (for healthy individuals). No more, no less!

On impulse I bought some of this bentonite clay. One pound was used to make a mudpack for my head held together by a plastic cap. The rest went into the bath. After soaking in the tub for twenty minutes and showering to rinse off the clay, I felt exhausted and lay down on the bed to rest, leaving the clay mess to be cleaned up later.

---

146 Check with your health professional before taking food supplements, herbs, or any other remedy or pharmaceutical medication. Combining prescription drugs with other remedies, herbs or food supplements may cause undesirable side effects. One older woman was diagnosed as having Alzheimer's disease and confined to a nursing home for three years before a physician discovered her memory problems were caused by heart medication. Keep in mind that "all-natural" does not mean that every natural substance is safe. Many all-natural remedies, herbs and pharmaceutical medications have dangerous side effects (*author*).

A Black Sticky Substance

When I returned hours later, the clay had settled to the bottom. Trying to avoid damaging the plumbing, I skimmed off the clear water and poured it down the sink, then scooped the remaining water/clay solution and carried it outside. I was astonished to find that the solid clay remaining in the bottom of the tub turned from a light tan/gray color into a black sticky tar-like substance. Wearing rubber gloves, I wrapped the toxic clay in crumpled newspaper and a heavy-duty garbage bag.

Amazed, I began sharing my experience with friends. One woman, also a victim of mercury poisoning, bought enough clay for her entire family. The residue from her four teenaged boys' baths was normal in color. Her husband's, however, left dark-colored sediment on the bottom of the tub. And my friend's results were like mine: black sticky stuff. (The clay has a particular affinity for mercury.)

Another friend suffering from mercury poisoning also took a clay bath, but forgot to wear rubber gloves when she cleaned up afterward (and got a chemical burn on her hand as she scooped up the clay).

Curious, I sent off a sample of my hair for analysis. The results showed no chemicals or metals present other than a small amount of aluminum. About five months later I took another clay bath. The clay came out normal in color, with only a few black specks in it. I knew without a doubt that the magical clay had done its work, saving my health and thousands of dollars.

Magical Clay

"Clay has been used for thousands of years and no one has been able to pin down what makes it a healer," observes Michael Abehera, author of *Amazing Cures from the Earth Itself—The Healing Clay.* Most users, he notes, seem content with the amazing results. But various observers offer different perspectives on how the clay works.

Raymond Dextreit, the French naturopath who popularized the clay cure in his own country, believes bentonite's powers transcend its purely three-dimensional physical properties. "From a thermodynamic point of view, clay cannot be the sole source of energy of the phenomenon it produces. Clay is a dramatic presence, a catalyst rather than an agent itself. This is possible because clay is alive."

Most of the poisons in the body Dextreit notes are positively charged, whereas clay has a negative electrical attraction. "These toxins cannot resist being drawn toward the clay."

Robert T. Martin, a mineralogist at MIT, points to bentonite's minute particles, which create a large surface area in proportion to the volume used. "The greater the surface area, the greater the power to pick up positively charged particles or toxins."

However one explains it, this natural earth remedy is a quick and inexpensive way to "pull" those toxic substances out of the body. Nevertheless, these are simple but important instructions that must be followed before and after the bath. It is also crucial to use "clean clay." We have tried numerous clays on the market and have found they have varied in results and uses. Most industrial clays (even many at health food stores) contain chemical emulsifiers, defeating the whole purpose of the bath, so please be selective in your choice of clay.

For more information on various clay detox bath kits formulated to assist in the removal of arsenic, aluminum, mercury, lead and various other environmental toxins, including those for exposure to radiation, contact 1-800-257-3315. There is also the Smoker's/Drug Detox Bath and the power of the New Energy Clay Bath (with very special clays). All information packets are free.

Lauana Lei is a world traveler, internationally recognized for her avid research and writing on health and environmental issues. She now resides in the Smoky Mountains of North Carolina.

Author's Note

The foregoing information was quoted in its entirety with permission from Lauana Lei. Since the article was written, a neutralizer has become available, which when applied after the bath, dissolves the clay so that it is safe to let the bath water flow down the drain. This author has no monetary connection to these products or to Ms. Lei. This information is presented because I believe these products are one of the easiest and least expensive ways to rid the body of mercury and environmental toxins. Remember that I am not a medical professional. If you have questions, do not take any action that makes you feel uncomfortable. Check with your physician or other medical professionals until you have enough accurate information to make a wise decision. In the final analysis, it is your pocketbook that pays the bill and it is you who must take the responsibility for your own decisions about your medical treatment plan.

Are there any cautions?

Yes! The mud bath is contraindicated if you have a heart condition, diabetes or high blood pressure. Check with your doctor beforehand if you are in a weakened health condition, take prescription medications, or are extremely toxic with chemicals/metals. Call the 800 numbers above for additional information. Do not take the detoxification bath until two hours after eating.

Pregnant women must not take hot baths, especially during mercury detoxification. If it is possible, a woman needs to have all of her mercury fillings replaced one year before becoming pregnant to prevent mercury from poisoning the fetus. If a woman does have mercury fillings, mercury from the mother's milk will poison her baby.

Epsom Salts Bath

Dr. Huggins recommends soaking in a hot bathtub at 104ºF for 20 minutes, just 20 minutes, not one degree higher or one minute longer than 20 minutes or you will heat the core temperature of your body too high. Cover yourself with a hot wet towel and place a wet hand towel over your head.

- The first two days add two cups of Epsom Salt to the bath water. Shower afterwards (SA).
- The third and fourth days add one-cup of Epsom Salt and one cup baking soda (SA).
- The fifth and sixth days add two cups baking soda to the bath water and add one pint of hydrogen peroxide to the bath water (SA). Your bath water may turn black. Repeat soak again in ten days, in two or three months and every six months for several years (SA).

Three problems I faced when soaking in the tub were to accurately determine the temperature of the bath water and to get the water high enough to cover my body. I solved the first two by purchasing a pool thermometer from a spa retailer and covering the tub drain with adhesive tape to allow hot water to completely cover my body. A cold tub will soak up heat faster than one might wish. Raising the water temperature to 107°F beforehand to heat the tub solved the third problem, allowing the water temperature to remain at 104°F for a longer period of time. Do not step into the water until the floating pool thermometer reads 104°F. Be sure to set the timer to ring at 20 minutes in case you fall asleep. Staying in the tub longer than 20 minutes will heat the core temperature of your body too high. Get out of the tub immediately when it rings.

Take these baths with caution if you are elderly or have any health concerns. Use a slightly lower temperature if 104°F seems too hot for you.

An Important Breakthrough

It is my personal view that any chelating agent causing mercury to be excreted through the intestinal track or kidneys should be avoided whenever possible. Some amount of mercury is reabsorbed from the feces by the liver and re-circulated throughout the whole body. Animal research at the University of Calgary entitled "Dental Mercury Impairs Kidney Function" concluded mercury produced a reduced rate of insulin clearance in urine consistent with impaired kidney function. Mercury poisoning and diabetes cause nephropathy, kidney failure. It seems safer to expel mercury directly through the skin. That aside, assuming the patient does not have too many mercury fillings,[147] there is a possibility the following information might be the breakthrough for which mercury-poisoned dental patients are searching.

I mentioned to Dr. Andrew Cutler, author of *Amalgam Illness: Diagnosis and Treatment,* that I had been diagnosed with kidney disease. He recommended Lipoic Acid (LA) to chelate mercury from my brain, liver and kidneys. I've been using LA for two weeks and cannot remember any time during the last 20 years I felt better than I do right now. My last test for kidney disease indicated that I must have been misdiagnosed. My hemoglobin A1C is 6.7 and I will get it lower. Below 7.0, microvascular damage caused by diabetes begins to reverse itself. Caution: stop eating flour products, rice or sugar in any form, and walk.

Natural Medicines Comprehensive Database, compiled by the editors of *Pharmacist's Letter's, 2000*, has this to say about Alpha Lipoic Acid: People use LA as an antioxidant, for diabetes, AIDS, cancer and liver conditions.

---

147 Dr. Huggins writes: after chelation, if the patient has mercury fillings in his or her mouth, mercury will return to previous levels within nine minutes

Journal of the American Society of Nephrology

Molecular Aspects of Lipoic Acid in the Prevention of Diabetes Complications

Department of Pharmacology and Toxicology, School of Pharmacy, University of Southern California, Los Angeles, California, USA; the BASF AG, Ludwigshafen, Germany; and the School of Food Biosciences, Hugh Sinclar Human Nutrition Unit, University of Reading, Reading, United Kingdom.

Abstract: a-Lipoic acid (LA) and its reduced form, dihydrolipoic acid, are powerful antioxidants. LA scavenges hydroxyl radicals, hypochlorous acid, peroxynitrite, and singlet oxygen. Dihydropoc acid also scavenges superoxide and peroxyl radicals and can regenerate thioredoxin, vitamin C, and glutathione, which in turn can recycle vitamin E. There are several possible sources of oxidative stress in diabetes including glycation reactions, decompartmentalization of transition metals, and the shift in the reduced-oxygen status of the diabetic cells. Diabetics have increased levels of lipid hydroperoxides, DNA adducts, and protein carbonylis. Available data strongly suggest that LA, because of its antioxidant properties, is particularly suited to the prevention and/or treatment of diabetic complications that arise from an overproduction of reactive oxygen and nitrogen species. In addition to its antioxidant properties, LA increases glucose uptake through recruitment of the glucose transporter-4 to plasma membranes, a mechanism that is shared with insulin-simulated glucose uptake. Further, recent trials have demonstrated that LA improves glucose disposal in patients with type II diabetes. In experimental and clinical studies, LA markedly reduced the symptoms of diabetic pathologies, including cataract formation, vascular damage, and polyneuropathy. To develop a better understanding of the preventive and therapeutic potentials of LA, much of the current interest is focused on elucidating in molecular mechanisms in redox dependent gene expression. Nutrition 2001; 17-888-895© Elsevier Science Inc. 2001

For the rest of the Story

Correction of sugar, fat and protein excesses and controlled supplementation of pyridoxine (vitamin B6), magnesium, chromium and coenzyme Q10 prevent diabetes and arteriosclerosis.

—Dr. John Ely

The 14-day average on my diabetes monitor today reads 99 mg/dl. It is higher than usual, because I had rice last night. Rice and potatoes have very high glycemic levels. Potatoes deposit glucose in the bloodstream faster than sugar. Excessive protein intake, e.g., meat, fish, cheese etc., further complicate kidney failure. When the level of urine in the bloodstream reaches 22 percent we die. An old military warhorse who dropped by several months ago told me he recovered from diabetes by eating nothing but salads and chicken. I never really liked salads, but became a greener immediately. Within a week or two I discovered that I enjoy salad.[148] My blood glucose levels dropped like a rock. I began to consume too much protein and noticed bubbles in the toilet water begin to look like a woman's bubble bath, a marker of kidney failure. Is this information important? You bet! It means most of us can recover from kidney disease. If we can just get dentists to discontinue the use of mercury amalgam and the public to stop consuming too much protein, fat, grain and junk food and sugar and walk, then diabetes, kidney disease and obesity will become insignificant medical problems.

---

148 Newman's Own Oil and Vinegar is the only salad dressing I use. It tastes great!

Speculation

I'm not supposed to hypothesize about treatment processes. On the other hand, the diagnosis of kidney failure is a disease I've not had time to work through yet. Too much information needs to reach the public about the toxicity of mercury amalgam dental fillings, root canals and cavitations to delay publishing any longer. Speaking for myself, I take two 100mg Alpha Lipoic Acid tablets, available over the counter in pharmacies or health food stores, three times a day for ten days, just ten days, and intend to repeat the regime every ten days until the bubbles in the toilet water disapear. Talk this over with your physician. This is new information and it is unlikely your doctor has had time to read the above research. For the person who has kidney failure, doing nothing is not an option.

Protocols for Allergy Testing

Dr. Theron Randolph's Protocol

At the time I was his patient (1982), Dr. Randolph had not recognized the connection between heavy metal poisoning, cerebral allergies and chronic disease. He taught us to discover which foods and chemicals produced brain-fog. He did send a few patients to the dentist, but in 1982 there was not enough information available to the medical community or to the public to grasp the issue.

We were fasted for approximately five days, sometimes longer, until the discharge from the alimentary canal was as clear as a glass of water. The nurse checked the toilet to make sure the patient did not cheat. At that point the patient becomes hypersensitive to food and chemicals. Dr. Randolph ordered our food from Mennonite farmers who had never chemicalized their soil. In some cases, when it was necessary, because a patient reacted to too many species of native animals, he ordered lion or hippopotamus meat from Africa. The first food I was tested on was cabbage. They gave me a whole head of steamed cabbage for lunch. I had only eaten perhaps a quarter of the head when there was a sudden burst of pain that felt like I'd laid my arm on an anvil and a blacksmith smashed my forearm with a two-pound hammer. It went down hill after that.

Looking at My Hospital Records, January 1982

"Cherries: (pulse) 86, 84, 86. Before: No symptoms. Full on 13 cherries—felt a switch in my head flick on—fuzz 1, mild headache .5, tired 2-20 min: stomach queasy—pain at bridge of nose, brain-fag—tired—feel lousy—went to sleep.

"Salmon: (pulse) 96, 99, 99, 99. Before, no symptoms—Could barely eat one and one half pieces of salmon-eating slowly—felt full. Pleased to feel stuffed on so little. 1 and 1/2 hours: Fuzz: brain-fog. Poor perception—tingling headache around eyes and frontal lobe.

"Pineapple: Before: (pulse) 86,90,90,90. (No reaction.)

"Removed books (from bedside table) yesterday—woke feeling best since being here. Opened book had an immediate cerebral reaction—headache—disorientation, confusion, sick, hungry. Did not feel... ." (The rest of the sentence is unintelligible because I couldn't write further.)

We were given all we desired of any one food. I cut the amount of the food I ordered two, maybe three times in 23 days. A petite physician patient, who had installed a new synthetic carpet in her office, developed brain-fag. She often ordered the same foods as I did. The food was excellent, but I gave her most of my servings, because I had lost my appetite. We laughed about the situation, because she probably weighed less than 105 pounds and at the time I weighed 278.[149]

Some physical and brain allergy reactions were extraordinarily painful and disorientating. One of the most terrifying incidents I felt was my reaction to formaldehyde. The incident is humiliating and painful to recall because I became totally disoriented. It was as if I had been frozen in space. Within ten seconds I could not move my fingers, turn my head, or call for assistance. I am surprised that I did not stop breathing. The nurse had turned and left the room. Eventually, a fellow passing in the hall glanced toward me and realized that I was in serious trouble. The nurse came running and someone administered oxygen. Oxygen usually stops allergic reactions. As someone spoke to me I could actually see the sound of their voice coming toward me in increments like death scenes in action movies.

---

149 I weigh 168.

These tests are not something to attempt by anyone except with a physician or a well-trained nurse in a hospital environmental allergy unit. One young woman had convulsions for two hours after eating one cherry. Dr. Randolph had a point system to indicate the severity of allergic reactions from 1 to 4. Four indicated the food or chemical provokes severe reactions. All brain allergies are number four. By testing enough foods, the staff is usually able to suggest a list of safe foods to rotate over a four-day period. Former allergy patients who were able to stick with the rotation diet became radiantly healthy within six months. In the beginning, when I was always spaced out and had so few free-foods, the plan was worthless for me.

Louise's job is exhausting and it is inconceivable to expect that she has the time to plan and cook special meals, but as I peruse my hospital records I realized that I am well enough and should have started Dr. Randolph's four-day rotation schedule years ago. I suspect the four-day rotation diet might put me over the top. I'd like my thought process to be as clear as some of the people I met over the years who stuck to the plan who are radiantly healthy. It's time to start cooking for myself.

Kinesiology: An Easy, Inexpensive Test

So, do I have a better solution for discovering foods that provoke physical disease and mental symptoms than Dr. Randolph's Provocative Challenge test? Perhaps.

Here Is How It Is Done

Asking a friend to help, extend your strongest arm directly out to your side and hold it in place. Do not peek as your friend inserts a cigarette or some other substance in your other hand. Have your friend face you so he is looking directly into your face. Neither one of you must smile or frown. Your friend should place his hand on your extended hand. His other hand should be placed on your opposite shoulder. He is to press on your hand. If the substance is good for you, your arm will lock in place. If you are sensitive to whatever substances you are holding, it does not take much pressure to cause your arm to drop. The easier it is to slide the hand down, the more sensitive you are to that particular item. Actually, I do not use my hand to push on the arm. I use my first two fingers. Heavily muscled men's arms will drop like an elevator if they are holding a substance toxic to them.

Although the above test is not as accurate as the Provocative Challenge test of Dr. Randolph's, it is good medicine. It's free, and for those who are temporarily broke, it is the only solution available. Even if you miss testing a few foods, discovering most foods to avoid and free foods that do not provoke brain-fog is a real plus.

Rotate free-foods over a four-day period. Do not eat the same food more often than once every four days or eventually you will become allergic to that food, too. Free-foods are like a bank account. Don't waste them.

For Alzheimer's Sufferers Fortunate Enough to Have Independent Means

A list of the physicians and mercury-free dentists can be found in Appendix IX. Do not bother them unless you intend to become their patient. All of them would like to talk with every single person suffering from heavy metal poisoning, but it is not possible. I spent over two years from early morning until late at night on the telephone talking with people who called me about Alzheimer's disease. One group of eight people flew in from Florida to seek information. Desperate husbands and wives drove long distances to show up on our doorstep. Piles of mail reached us from five to 14 inches high and sometimes higher, every other day for more than a year. Our hearts went out to all those people, but it became impossible to continue such a hectic pace. We moved and changed our unlisted telephone number a half-dozen times before life began to return to normal. Four years later, physicians and local Alzheimer's Association secretaries told me they still received calls for me from people who wanted more information. I wish that we could have afforded to help everyone who asked, but it was impossible. We estimate that it cost our family a minimum of ten times more than I earned from *Beating Alzheimer's* to help these people. I expect it could, if I allow it to happen, turn out to be a similar story with this book, but I need to get back to work. We lost my income after I developed Alzheimer's disease. I'm 71. It's time to pay off the mortgage so Louise can safely retire after I die. Louise has paid the bills for almost 20 years. She is tired. She needs a break. It is my turn to earn a paycheck. Physicians face a similar challenge. Knowledge and time are their working capital and no matter how unjust it seems to the caller, doctors have to be paid for their time. There isn't any other way they can afford to stay in business. In addition, the physicians and clinics I refer to have patients stacked up all over the place waiting to be seen. Be considerate; please do not waste their time.

The only thing left to do is to remind the Alzheimer's sufferer, if the conditions exist that allow you to rotate free-foods every four days, do it. You will recover faster. Not only that, over several months you will regain the vitality missing in your life. Now, get yourself out of the easy chair and go for a walk. If you can't walk, crawl around the house or sit on a trampoline and bounce until you regain enough energy and strength to stand, then walk.

Recovery does not go in a straight line. You will fall off the wagon now and then, or inadvertently expose yourself to chemicals or substances in foods that temporarily cause you to feel miserable. Maybe your pillow will become too full of dust mites, etc., etc. But stick with the plan. You will be glad you did.

A Personal View

If I am inadvertently exposed to massive doses of malodorous chemicals, I become befuddled or the fumes provoke explosive irrational behavior. Pork and minute amounts of out-gassing newspaper ink cause me to fall asleep. MSG (monosodium glutamate) hurts worse than a mean hangover (I do not drink). The only reason I am well is that I have learned which substances provoke brain-fog and brain-fag in my immediate environment and either neutralize the offending substance with plants or air filters, move the offending item away from me, or move me away from it. It takes a while to learn how to deal with the problem. It requires constant vigilance and in a way, it's a pain in the neck. Of course, if I had not learned how to live in my environment, I would not be complaining. I would be in an insane asylum, prison or would have died from Alzheimer's disease ten or 15 years ago.

Although none of this information on heavy metal toxicity and food/chemical allergies is well understood by the traditional psychiatric community, law enforcement agencies, the legal profession or the prison system, these substances can and do provoke erratic behavior and intense hostility. Keep in mind that I am talking about law-abiding citizens who have become mentally ill and entangled with the law, not professional criminals. These substances are also one of the underlying causes of dysfunctional family relationships that produce neurosis through generations of offspring. I could give many examples of brain-fag related to alcoholism, assault and even murder. I have watched schizophrenic mental patients, men with real character, make excellent progress in overcoming their illness until they inadvertently ate foods or drank alcohol or used shaving lotion that turned them from Dr. Jekyll to Mr. Hyde as fast as flipping a light switch. In that state, they might just as well have been on Jupiter, and there wasn't the slightest doubt that if I had provoked any of them they would have murdered me without the slightest hesitation.

In summary, the three points I am trying to make are that most foods, especially favorite foods, chemicals, pharmaceuticals, herbs and odors, have both positive and negative side effects. The second point is that "brain allergy" is the missing piece of the schizophrenia or Alzheimer's puzzle that psychiatrists and neurologists do not understand. The third is that the underlying cause of brain allergy is heavy metal poisoning, mainly from mercury amalgam dental fillings. Other sources of mercury are fish, gold-mining operations, thermometers and machine shops. Mercury is used in the pharmaceutical, chemical and manufacturing industries. It is found in 4,000 products.

NAMI and the Drug Companies

The National Advocates for the Mentally Ill (NAMI) receives huge donations from multi-national drug companies. The reason? Money. Most mercury-toxic patients displaying atypical behavior are misdiagnosed as having endogenous depression, schizophrenia, dementia or Alzheimer's disease and given prescriptions for psychotropic medications while the primary cause of schizophrenia, mercury poisoning and jawbone infection, is ignored.

According to material obtained by Mother Jones, 18 drug firms gave NAMI a total of $11.72 million between 1996 and mid-1999. These include:

$2.08 million	Janssen
$1.87 million	Pfizer
$1.24 million	Abbott Lab.
$658,000	Wyeth-Ayerst Phar.
$613,505	Bristol-Meyers Squibb

NAMI's largest contributor in the State of Washington is Eli Lilly:

$5,000	Astra Zeneca
$91,000	Eli Lilly
$18,200	Janssen
$6,000	Novatis
$5,000	Pfizer
$5,000+	Zenica

Total: $130,200 donated to NAMI Washington from January 6, 1998 to February 15, 2000 (26 months).

Scientist's Death Traced to Seemingly Trifling Mishap

HELEN O'NEIL, Associated Press
Sunday, September 14, 1997, Seattle Times

Tiny drop of mercury spilled in chemistry lab proves deadly

Lyme, New Hampshire - It was just a drop of liquid, just a tiny glistening drop. It glided over her glove like a jewel. Scientist Karen Wetterhahn knew the risks: the bad stuff kills if you get too close.

She took all the normal precautions working with mercury in her Dartmouth University laboratory wearing protective gloves and eye goggles, working under a ventilated hood that sucks up chemical fumes.

So on that sunny day in August, when she accidentally spilled a drop, she didn't think anything of it. She washed her hands, cleaned her instruments and went home.

It was just a drop of liquid, just a tiny glistening drop.

At first, friends thought she had caught a stomach bug on her trip to Malaysia. It wasn't until she started bumping into doors that her husband, Leon Webb, began to worry. Karen, always so focused, always so sure of her next step, was suddenly falling down as if she were drunk. In fifteen years together she had never been sick, never stopped working, never complained. Leon was stunned when she called for a ride home from work.

A few nights later Leon drove her to the emergency room. It was Monday, January 20, 1997, five months since she had spilled the drop in the lab.

Just a single drop of liquid, yet somehow it had penetrated her skin. By the weekend, Karen couldn't walk, her speech was slurred and her hands trembled. The initial diagnosis of "virus" seemed awfully vague for symptoms that were getting worse every day.

"It's mercury poisoning," Dr. David Nierenberg said. "We have to start treatment immediately." Leon hung up with relief. At last, they understood the problem. Now maybe they could fix it.

It seemed impossible to believe anything could be wrong with Karen Wetterhahn, one of those quietly impressive individuals whose lives seemed charmed from the start. Serious and hardworking, she excelled at everything she turned to: science, sailing or skiing.

Karen was always the brilliant one of the family, the one who would do great things. And she did, becoming the first woman chemistry professor at Dartmouth, running a world-renowned laboratory on chromium research. It was important work, the kind that could lead to cures for cancer and AIDS. Karen thrived on it.

At home, she would throw great neighborhood parties by the pool, or gather up the family and drag them off to the golf course, or the tennis court, or a kid's hockey game.

"We never knew she was a world famous scientist," one neighbor said afterward. "She was just Char and Ashley's mom."

Mercury poisoning. Karen beamed when she heard the news. Finally, something she understood. Something she could explain. They would feed her fat white nasty-tasting pills that would flush the poison out of her system. Science would cure her, she told her husband, giddy with excitement as she sat in bed surrounded by her children and her notes.

Back in January, virtually nothing was known about the extraordinary dangers of dimethylmercury, the rare man-made compound Karen had spilled. Scientists didn't know it could seep through a latex glove like a drop of water through a Kleenex. Doctors didn't know it could break down the body over the course of a few months, slowly, insidiously and irreversibly.

Above all, no one knew how to stop its deadly progress, as it cut off her hearing, her speech, her vision, reducing her body to a withered shell. Today, because of Karen, the world knows so much more.

Quicksilver, as mercury is called, has long played a sinister game of seduction with science. One of the world's oldest metals, it comes in various forms: some that heal, some that kill. Dimethylmercury, a colorless liquid that looks like water but is three times heavier, is far more toxic than other forms, the kind used in thermometers and batteries and medicine. It's made purely for research and is rarely used.

There was only one documented case of dimethylmercury poisoning this century, a Czech chemist in 1972 who had suffered the same symptoms as Karen and died. A handful of people had been exposed directly to pure methylmercury, another toxic mercury compound, and died. There was no telling if dimethylmercury would act the same way.

Karen herself was beginning to understand. There was a desperate look on her face as she pointed to the clock when it was time to take her pills. Still, she kept up a brave face, kept saying not to worry.

That was Jan. 31, 1997, three days after the diagnosis. A week later, Karen was transferred to Massachusetts General Hospital for a massive blood transfusion that nearly killed her.

Leon was pacing at home again, torn between honoring his wife's wish not to alert her parents and the feeling that she was sinking faster than she knew.

The phone rang. The nurse said Karen wanted to talk to her son, Ashley. From her hospital bed, the mother struggled. She drooled and moaned and the words just wouldn't come. Ashley, 14, waited uncomfortably. He didn't like the silence. "Hi, mom" he coaxed loud so she might hear. It was useless. The nurse ended the torture and took the phone. "She just wanted to say goodnight," Ashley says, bowing his head to hide the tears when he remembers the last time he talked to his mother. "She couldn't even say goodnight."

Others remember final moments, too, although everything was happening so fast that they didn't seem like good-byes at the time. But friends could see the toll on the scientist's mind and body. They could see her faith fading, even as she continued to talk about being back on her feet for her new spring course. The day the ambulance came to take her to Massachusetts, she cried uncontrollably.

Karen's lab was shut down. Her family, students and co-workers were tested. Her hospital room was checked for airborne mercury from her breath. Federal environmental and health agencies were alerted, as was the state health department. Her car and clothes and house were sniffed with mercury-detectors.

Scientists and doctors around the world offered their services. "It was an extraordinary outpouring," Nierenberg says.

But Karen was slipping too fast to appreciate it. Ten days after the diagnosis, on February 7th, she fell into a coma. Leon told the doctors he was taking her home. Back at Dartmouth Hitchcock Hospital, her family kept vigil by the bedside, her parents and sister talking to her as her body thrashed and moaned.

Just a tiny drop of poison and she was fighting it with all her might. It became too difficult for the children to visit. Even friends stayed home, waiting for the phone call that would tell them it was over.

Her husband stroked her face. Her sister and her best friend washed her hair. Doctors tried treatments never attempted on humans before. But they couldn't save her from the poison. June 8th, it took her life. "She didn't suffer," Ashley told his eighth-grade class the next day. "She just stopped breathing."

It was 10 months since she had spilled the drop in the lab, four months after she had slipped into a coma.

While she could still speak, she urged doctors and scientists to learn everything they could from her accident and to warn the world about the dangers. The world has already learned that the gloves that were supposed to protect her actually acted as a conductor to the poison. It learned that dimethylmercury, so easy to order in research catalogs, is more deadly than anyone had imagined. Saddest of all, it learned that by the time the symptoms showed, it was too late.

Her funeral took place on a hot summer day to the strains of a flute and a choir singing "Be Not Afraid." In the packed college chapel, the sense of betrayal was as powerful as the sense of loss. Colleagues wept as they eulogized a modern-day Madame Curie who had sacrificed her life to her cause.

Alone and bewildered, Leon sat in the front pew, looking out of place in his dark funeral suit, tears streaming down his face. It all seemed like a dream, he says later. "No," he corrects himself, "a nightmare. She loved her work," he said. "It made her happy."

She couldn't have known the risks. She couldn't have known how bad the stuff really was. No one knew.

Just a tiny drop of liquid, sweet-smelling, dense and deadly.

Legalities and Legislation

ADA And CDA Sued For Deceiving Patients About Mercury Amalgam Dental Fillings

Press Release: Los Angeles, California, 06/12/01 - The American Dental Association and its California affiliate were sued today in California Superior Court for their unlawful practice of deceiving patients about the presence of mercury in the most widely used type of dental fillings. The case charges the ADA and its largest state affiliate with deceiving consumers into thinking amalgam fillings are made of silver, when in fact the major component is 50 percent mercury. Only about 19 percent of a mercury amalgam filling is composed of silver.

The lawsuits were filed this morning by public interest attorneys Shawn Khorrami of Los Angeles and Charles G. Brown of Washington, D.C. on behalf of organizations and individuals active in the effort to end the use of mercury in dental amalgam fillings.

In addition to filing the lawsuits, the attorneys served 60 days notice (as required by law) that they intend to sue the ADA under the provisions of Proposition 65, the anti-toxics measure passed by California voters in 1986. Under Prop. 65, the State of California has identified mercury as a chemical known to be a reproductive and/or developmental toxin.

The California Dental Board did everything they could to ignore Proposition 65. Finally: The California Legislature voted 70 to 1 to disband their entire Dental Board as of December 31, 2001. When Governor Gray Davis fired all of them, he said the dental board was working for the ADA, not in the interests of dental patients.

"It is long past time for the ADA and the CDA to 'open wide' and start using the 'M' word," said Brown, the former West Virginia state Attorney General who is the lead attorney for the national legal battle against mercury in dental fillings. "Mercury is universally recognized as an extremely dangerous toxin. One filling contains 750 milligrams of mercury, enough to contaminate a small lake. The ADA is out of the medical mainstream in claiming that mercury is safe for use in human beings."

Maine Passes Legislation Guaranteeing Accurate Patient Information on Mercury Amalgam Filling Toxicity

Augusta, Maine, 08/23/2001

Governor Angus King today signed the most advanced bill in the United States requiring dentists to inform their patients that amalgam dental fillings contain a large percentage of the toxic element mercury, which can be harmful to the wearer's health.

In his preliminary remarks before signing the bill, Governor King noted that Maine has probably taken more action to get mercury out of the air and water than any other state in the union. "And yet we all carry it around in our mouths," he remarked. Senate President Michael Michaud spearheaded the bill and Representatives Joanne Twoomey and Steven Stanley, all of whom were present, spoke at the signing. Consumer advocates Pam Anderson and Dr. Tom Anderson, a mercury-free dentist from Houlton, Maine, who led grassroots support for the bill, participated in the ceremony as well. Senate President Michaud cited the courage of the many individuals who testified on behalf of the bill, especially the dentists who came forward to endorse it despite the opposition of the American Dental Association.

"We hope that the U.S. will take Maine's lead and move forward with legislation at the national level," he said.

The bill mandates that every dentist's office will feature a poster and a brochure informing patients about the presence of mercury in amalgam fillings and about its negative health effects. Scientific research has shown that dental amalgam is the chief source of mercury in the human body. For that reason Rep. Twoomey described the bill as a major step forward for women of childbearing age and for children, who receive their first exposure to mercury in the womb and from their mother's breast milk. Mercury has been implicated in neurological disorders of children such as autism and ADD/ADHD, and in fertility problems in women.

"We are delighted that this bill has been signed," said Rep. Stanley. "It is a major step forward to protect the health of Maine citizens." Pam Anderson added that the group hopes Maine's next step would be to ban the use of dental amalgam in all women of childbearing age and in children.

Other participants in the press conference were Kathleen McGee, Director of the Maine Toxic Action Coalition; Maine DAMS (Dental Amalgam Mercury Syndrome) Coordinator Marjorie Monteleone, and New Hampshire DAMS Coordinator Rosie Cronen; representatives from the Maine People's Alliance, the Maine Citizens for Affordable Health Care, and the Maine Department of Environmental Protection; Dr. Gerald Vermette, a mercury-free dentist; Rosemary Fecteau, Ph.D., whose husband died of mercury toxicity from his dental fillings; Charles Brown, attorney for the national organization Consumers for Dental Choice; and New York City DAMS Coordinator Dr. Lydia Bronte, author of a widely respected book, *The Mercury In Your Mouth. The Truth About "Silver" Dental Fillings.*

"The public is being deceived by the terminology used for these fillings," said Charles Brown in his remarks. "The ADA calls them 'silver' fillings, but they are really mercury fillings. If people knew the principal ingredient is mercury, they would not want these fillings in their teeth."

Governor King compared the current use of mercury in dental fillings with the 1950's use in shoe stores of powerful x-ray machines called fluoroscopes, which exposed hundreds of thousands of adults and children to high doses of toxic x-rays. "Every child who went into the shoe store to buy new shoes would put his feet into the fluoroscope so the bones could be seen," Governor King recalled. "People who worked in the store were exposed to the radiation all day; children played games around the machine. Now we realize it was a terrible thing to do, but then it seemed perfectly normal. Some day we will wonder how we could ever have put such a toxic substance into the human mouth."

STATE OF NEW HAMPSHIRE

In the Year of Our Lord Two Thousand Two
AN ACT relative to the use of mercury amalgam fillings by dentists.
Be it Enacted by the Senate and House of Representatives in General Court convened:

96:1 New Subdivision; Mercury Amalgam. Amend RSA 317-A by inserting after section 37 the following new subdivision:

Mercury Amalgam

317-A: 38 Mercury Amalgam Information.
A dentist shall present patients having dental restorative procedures with a standardized pamphlet developed by the board in consultation with the department of health and human services regarding the risks and benefits of dental materials, including mercury amalgam, and shall discuss with the patient the choices of restorative dental materials prior to their use.

96:2 New Paragraph; Mercury Amalgam; Information. Amend RSA 126-A:3 by inserting after paragraph V the following new paragraph:
VI. The department shall provide information to the citizens of New Hampshire, within its existing resources, about the risks and benefits of dental restorative materials including the use of amalgam in children under the age of 6.

96:3 New Paragraph; Environmental Services; Mercury Amalgams. Amend RSA 485-A:4 by inserting after paragraph XVII the following new paragraph:

XVIII. To establish rules for dental offices relative to the use of environmentally appropriate disposal equipment for amalgam waste to trap and dispose of mercury.

96:4 New Paragraph; Rulemaking. Amend RSA 485-A:6 by inserting after paragraph XII the following new paragraph:

XIII. The disposal of dental office waste under RSA 485-A:4, XVIII.
96:5 Effective Date. This act shall take effect January 1, 2003.

Approved: May 3, 2002)
(Effective Date: January 1, 2003)

Oregon Dental Board Rescinds Gag Rule

March 8, 2002, the Oregon Dental Board voted unanimously to rescind a rule that has been on their books since 1990 that effectively gagged dentists from discussing the potentially harmful effects of mercury exposure emanating from mercury-amalgam dental fillings. The issue was brought to a head by the ACLU protesting to the State Attorney General that the dental board's rule was a clear violation of a dentist's right to free speech under the U.S. and Oregon constitutions.

For More Information

Physicians and Dentists

Telephone numbers, Web sites and mailing addresses change over the years. Researchers, doctors and dentists retire. The information below is accurate at publication and hopefully will be available for many years. Later on it may be necessary for the reader to contact several telephone numbers or Web sites to obtain the information the reader is seeking. I regret that it is impossible for me to accept telephone calls or answer mail anymore. I found working one-on-one to be far more expensive, stressful and time-consuming than the public realizes. Public speaking to large audiences, radio or television shows is a more productive use of my energy and time. I will accept speaking engagements in any university[150] or country in the world.

DAMS: A wealth of information can be obtained from DAMS (Dental Amalgam Mercury Syndrome). They should be able to locate mercury-free dentists and physicians in your area who understand mercury toxicity. Patients may contact DAMS for Information Packets. DAMS' web page is one of the most important sites on the Internet for accurate information about mercury toxicity and the healing process. Web site: http://www.amalgam.org. Address: DAMS INC., P.O. Box 7249, Minneapolis, MN, 55407. Telephone (800) 311-6265.

150 I believe in our young people. University students are the world's next generation of informed leaders and are quick to recognize deception. It is unlikely that I will live long enough to stop dentists from placing mercury amalgam dental fillings or doing root canals. But, dentists are going to have a heck of a time doing business as usual once our young people become informed.

Jonathan Collin, MD: nutritional medicine and chelation specialist, editor of the Townsend Letter for Doctors and Patients, 911 Tyler Street, Port Townsend, WA 98368-6541, http://www.tldp.com/.

Sandra Denton, MD: There are many competent dentists and physicians who treat chronic disease in the United States and elsewhere whom I do not know well enough to recommend. A physician in the United States that I do recommend is Dr. Sandra Denton, the director of the Alaska Alternative Medicine Clinic in Anchorage, Alaska, (907) 563-6200.

Dr. Boyd Haley: Dr. Haley is Chair of the Department of Chemistry, University of Kentucky. One of the best web sites for medical professionals about the mercury-amalgam issue is http://www.altcorp.com. Dr. Haley's credentials are impeccable and he is as knowledgeable about the amalgam and root canal issues as anyone in the United States.

Hal Huggins, DDS: If I was looking for a dentist, the first thing I would do is go to http://www.hugnet.com and read all the information Dr. Huggins has to offer. Dr. Hal Huggins' telephone number in the United States is (719) 522-0566 or 888-843-5832.

Thomas Rau, DDS: Another physician I know by reputation is Dr. Thomas Rau, medical director of the Paracelsus Clinic in Lüstmuhle, Switzerland. Their telephone number from the United States is 011-41-71-335-71-71. In other countries the only numbers that change are the "long-distance code" itself, e.g., someone from Brazil or the Soviet Union would substitute 011 with their own long-distance code. The receptionist speaks German fluently and, with some difficulty, understands English.

Tom Warren: http://www.beatingchronicdisease.com

Well Mind Association: Their address is 4649 Sunnyside Avenue North, Room 344, Seattle WA 98013 USA; telephone (206) 547-6167, Web address http://www.speakeasy.org/~wma. The WMA newsletter gave me the first clue pointing to dental amalgam as being the source of my distress.

Dental Materials Biocompatibility Blood Testing Facilities

Peak Energy: Telephone (800) 331-2303 or (719) 548-1600. Their Web address is http:/www.peakenergy.com.

Clifford Consulting and Research: Telephone (719) 550-0008. Their Web address is http://www.ccrlab.com.

To Locate Orthomolecular Physicians:

Matrix, Inc. provides physician referrals: Telephone (1-719-522-0566). Address P.O. Box 49145, Colorado Springs, Colorado 80949-9145.

Equipment

Dust and/or Pollen Respirator:

Mine Safety Appliances: Telephone 1 (800) MSA-2222 from anywhere in the U.S. including Alaska and Hawaii.

The filters I purchased, Dust Foe 66 and Dust Foe 77, are not manufactured anymore, but MSA probably has the best dust and pollen filters in the marketplace. Choose a lightweight easy-to-care-for model. Flowers and odoriferous trees and shrubs, at least in me, cause muddled thought process. Scotch Broom is particularly obnoxious.

Air Filters:

The Sharper Image Ionic Breeze 1 (800) 344-4444

Water testing:

National Testing Laboratory 1 (800) 458-3330

Whole House Water Filters:

Coast Filtration, Inc. 1 (800) 542-6723

The Mercury Vapor Analyzer:

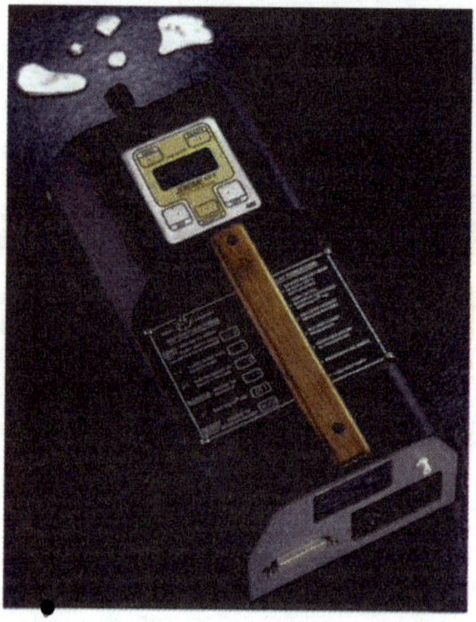

The Jerome® 431-X Mercury Vapor Analyzer uses a global film sensor for the detection and accurate measurement of toxic mercury vapor in the air.

It is designed to give accurate readings of mercury vapor out-gassing from the dental patient's mercury amalgam fillings.

A portable hand-held unit, the Jerome 431-X can easily be carried to locations of mercury concerns. Simple, push-button operation allows users to measure mercury levels in just seconds. The range of the 431-X is from 0.000 to 0.999 mg/m3 Hg. The gold film sensor is inherently stable and selective to mercury, eliminating interference common to ultraviolet analyzers, such as water vapor and hydrocarbons.

The 431-X includes features not available in older Jerome models. When attached to either a data logger or computer, the analyzer automatically regenerates the sensor when it becomes saturated and then resumes sampling. An improved film regeneration circuit makes the sensor last even longer.

For more information on the Jerome 431-X, contact a technical sales representative at 800-528-7411 or 602-470-1414.

A short bibliography for those who do not have access to the Internet.

Dr. Russell Blaylock, *Excitotoxins: The Taste that Kills*, Health Press, Santa Fe, NM, 1994.

Dr. Mark Breiner, *Whole Body Dentistry*, Quantum Press, Fairfield, CT, 06432, 1999.

Dr. Lydia Bronte, *The Mercury In Your Mouth: The Truth About "Silver" Dental Fillings*, Quicksilver Press, 1997.

Andrew H. Cutler, PhD, *Amalgam Illness: Diagnosis and Treatment*, Self-published 1999. Telephone 949-857-0410.

Dr. Janette D. Sherman, *Chemical Exposure and Disease: The Professional and Layperson's Guide To Understanding, Cause and Effect* (between chemical exposure and disease-author), Princeton Scientific Publishing Company, Inc. Princeton, NJ, 08543, 1994.

Debra Lynn Dadd, *Home Safe Home: Protecting Yourself and Your Family from Everyday Toxics and Harmful Household Products in the Home*, Putnam, New York, 1997.

Lono Kahuna Dupua Ao, *Don't Drink the Water: A guide to understanding and resolving our problem with contaminated drinking water*, Kali Press, Box 2169, Pagosa Springs, CO, 81147, May 1996.

Dr. Hal Huggins, *It's All in Your Head: The Link Between Amalgam Fillings and Illness*, Avery, New York, NY, 1993.

Dr. Hal Huggins and Dr. Thomas Levy, MD, *Uninformed Consent: The Hidden Dangers of Dental Care*, Hampton Roads, Charlottesville, VA, 22902, 1999.

Bonnye Matthews, *Chemical Sensitivity: A Guide to Coping with Hypersensitivity Syndrome, Sick Building Syndrome and other Environmental Illnesses*, McFarland & Company, Inc., Jefferson, NC, and London, 1992.

Dr. George Meinig, *The Root Canal Cover-Up: A Founder of the Association of Root Canal Specialists Discovers Evidence That Root Canals Damage Your Health-Learn What to Do*, Bion Publishing, Ojai, CA, 1994.

Dr. Abram Hoffer and Dr. Morton Walker, *Smart Nutrients: A Guide to Nutrients That Can Prevent and Reverse Senility*, Avery, New York NY 1997.

Dr. Francis Pottenger Jr., *Pottenger's Cats: A Study in Nutrition*, Price-Pottenger Nutrition Foundation, P.O. Box 2614, La Mesa, CA 92004, 1983.

Dr. Laura Newman, *Make Your Juicer Your Drug Store*, Benedict Lust Publications, New York, NY, 10156.

Dr. Weston Price, *The Price of Root Canals* (compiled by Hal Huggins) is available through the Price-Pottenger Nutrition Foundation, P.O. Box 2614, La Mesa, CA 92004 (619) 462-7600.

Dr. Weston Price, *Nutrition and Physical Degeneration*, Keats Publishing, Canaan, Connecticut, 1938, republished in1998.

Dr. Theron Randolph, *Alternative Approach to Allergies: The New Field of Environmental Medicine that Unravels the Causes of Mental and Physical Ills* is available through the Price-Pottenger Foundation, your book dealer, www.amazom.com, or found in a public library.

Dr. Janette Sherman, *Chemical Exposure and Disease, The Professional and Lawperson's Guide to Understanding Cause and Effect* (between chemical exposure and disease-author), Princeton Scientific Publishing, Princeton, NJ 1994.

Tom Warren, *Beating Alzheimer's*, Penguin Putnam, East Rutherford, NJ, 1989.

Alternative Medicine: Everything one must know about effective therapies and affordable self-help cures. A definitive guide compiled by Burton Goldberg. Future Medicine Publishing Inc., 1640 Blvd., Suite # 2, Tiburon, CA, 94920.

Suffice it to say that I downloaded almost a six-foot stack of mercury research papers off the Internet pertaining to the amalgam issue. I probably read three times that many, and more than 40 books on health and nutrition as well as the mercury amalgam issue during the last eight years this book has been in progress. One new book that I should mention is *Amalgam Illness: Diagnosis and Treatment* by Dr. Andrew H. Cutler. His book is stapled to avoid out-gassing formaldehyde fumes found in glue that binds the book cover to the manuscript. Stapling may not look professional, but it is more expensive than gluing on the cover. I had the first edition of *Beating Alzheimer's* stapled together and it was criticized for looking cheap and unprofessional. When Avery published the second edition, they were able to find glue without formaldehyde and printed the second edition of *Beating Alzheimer's* with vegetable dye instead of petrochemical ink that out-gasses hydrocarbon fumes (causing sleep, brain-fog and/or irritability in sensitive individuals). This information probably seems absurd to those who are not chemically sensitive, especially when students and librarians are exposed to thousands of books for years on end, but when I was first diagnosed with Alzheimer's disease, it was impossible to visit a library without developing brain-fog from out-gassing chemicals.

These two books, *Beating Alzheimer's* and *Amalgam Illness: Diagnosis and Treatment,* are the only reading material safe to leave in the bedroom. Even after two decades, I rarely read newspapers or new magazines in the house. My wife sometimes reads at the kitchen table, but Louise never allows printed material to accumulate because outgassing hydrocarbon fumes from new printed material cause me to become obnoxious.

Purchasing Books

Most of the above books can be obtained from the Price-Pottenger Foundation, (619) 462-7600, (800) 366-3748 or buy them through your local bookstore.

Summary

If Alzheimer's sufferers have enough cognition to understand the messages in these books, they will learn more about the cause of their distress and know more about how to recover their short-term memory than most of their dentists and physicians.

The trick is not in reading these things—it is in action! It is in doing it! Fan open the pages and air out all books not printed with non-toxic ink for at least two weeks outside of the house before anyone suffering short-term memory loss attempts to read them. For the first several weeks I would prefer readers not to read anything except this book, *Reversing Chronic Disease*, and to begin a regular walking program. It is too confusing for the Alzheimer's sufferer to put everything together all at once. For starters, stick with Chapter III and walk until you begin to feel stronger while your thought process clears.

Internet Links

It is prudent to update your anti-virus program.

Anti-Amalgam Links

Affinity Labeling Technologies: http://www.altcorp.com

BBC Online: http://www.bbc.co.uk/health/teeth/dentme.shtml

BioProbe: dedicated to providing you with the most current and accurate information available on the potential health effects of ''silver'' dental fillings. Web site for Sam Ziff and Dr. Michael Ziff, author of many books on mercury amalgams: http://www.bioprobe.com/faq.asp

Can Mercury-Silver Fillings Cause Disease? http://webm63bb.ntx.net/can.htm

Capital University School of Integrated Medicine:

http://www.cuim.edu

Cavitat MedicalTechnologies, Inc.:

http://cavitatmedtech.homestead.com/index.html

Chronic Illness and Chronic Mercury Exposure from Amalgams and the Environment: http://www.ephca.com/ci&cme.htm

Citizens for Health: http://www.citizens.org/AlternativeMedicine/CDCP/dental.htm

Clifford Materials Reactivity Testing: http://www.ccrlab.com

Common questions/answers regarding mercury amalgams: Questions and Answers concerning the Dental Materials in your mouth and your health! Are the silver fillings in your teeth REALLY silver? http://www.sukel.com/merc-qa.htm

Condensed from an article by Dr. Thomas Levy of Colorado Springs, Colorado (Extraordinary Science, April-June 1994): http://www.consultclarity.com/blazing/dental.html

DAMS (Dental Amalgam Mercury Syndrome): a non-profit organization dedicated to public education about the health hazards associated with common dental practices; http://www.amalgam.org

Dangers of Amalgam (Mercury) Fillings: http://www.nccn.net/~wwithin/amalgam.htm

Dental Danger-by Tony Copple: In the last few years, evidence has come to light of the dangers of significant toxicity that most people have in their own mouths as a result of dental work with mercury amalgam: http://www.ncf.carleton.ca/~aj624/dental.html

Dental Health Associates: http://membrane.com/philanet/dentist/detox.html

Dental Research: http://www.geocities.com/ResearchTriangle/2888/research.html

Dentistry and the Environment (internal and external): http://www.envirodental.co.uk

DMPS Backfire: http://www.dmpsbackfire.com

Effects of Mercury Poisoning in Humans:

http://danpatch.ecn.purdue.edu/~epados/mercury/pano/src/effects.htm

Environ news by topic: Mercury Toxicity: http://ehis.niehs.nih.gov/topic/heavymetal.html

Evidence Linking Silver-Mercury Fillings to Alzheimer's disease: by

Kip Sullivan, JD;
http://www.lightparty.com/Health/SilverFillings.html

Forty scientific abstracts (conducted in 1995):
http://www.algonet.se/~leif/OldAbr95.html

Dr. Hal Huggins and his official site for information:
http://www.hugnet.com/

Holistic Dental Association: http://www.holisticdental.org

Dr. Hulda Clark talks with Dr. Frank Jerome about cleaning up your dentalware: http://www.consultclarity.com/blazing/dentalware.html

IAOMT Amalgam Removal Protocol: Covers amalgam removal protocols and detoxification; http://www.holisticmed.com/dental/amalgam/iaomt.txt

International Academy of Oral Medicine and Toxicology:
http://www.iaomt.org/

Mercury amalgam safety: rethinking dangerous decisions. Article by Dr. Zoltan P. Rona:
http://www.selene.com/healthlink/amalgam.html

Mercury Amalgam-A Hazardous Material:
http://pages.prodigy.com/cent4dent/mercury.htm

Mercury and Amalgams: http://dmoz.org/Health/Alternative/Non-Toxic_Living/Mercury_and_Amalgams

Mercury Controversy: http://www.u-net.com/four-d/mercury.htm

Mercury fact sheet: http://www.geocities.com/Yosemite/Rapids/6464/hg_dyk.html

Mercury Free and Healthy, The Dental Amalgam Issue: Prepared December 1998 by DAMS Inc. along with Consumers for Dental Choice. A Project of the National Institute for Science, Law and Public Policy,

1424 16th Street, NW Suite 105, Washington, D.C. 20036; http://www.amalgam.org

Mercury in Saliva Study: http://www.uni-tuebingen.de/KRAUSS/amalgam.html

Mercury in Tooth: http://www.geocities.com/TelevisionCity/Station/6000/

Mercury Study Report to Congress: http://www.epa.gov/ttn/uatw/112nmerc/mercover.html

Mercury toxicity advice from a dentist: http://pages.prodigy.com/cent4dent

More facts about the dangers of mercury-amalgam fillings: Amalgam-Related Illness, Frequently Asked Questions (FAQ). An excellent site maintained by Leif Hedegard: http://www.algonet.se/~leif/AmFAQigr.html

Online Dental Injury Community and Search Engine: http://web-maker.com/dihi/index.html

Peak Energy Performance (materials reactivity Testing): http://www.peakenergy.com/

Preventive Dental Health Association: An excellent source of information about the hazards of mercury and fluoride. One section carefully refutes pro-amalgam statements made by the ADA; http://emporium.turnpike.net/P/PDHA/health.htm

Report on the 50-State Petition: http://www.swankin-turner.com/status.html

Tom Warren: http://www.beatingchronicdisease.com

Works of Dr. Edward C. Rosenow: http://www.angelfire.com/ca/instituteofscience/rosenow.html

Swedish Association of Dental Mercury Patients: http://www.tf.nu/indexeng-2.html

Thinking Person's Guide To Perfect Health Dental Amalgam Mercury Poisoning: This is an excellent website, except for one mistake (considering this paper was written in 1996, it is understandable). If the patient has any sort of mental problem, forget the information about DMPS. I do agree that just one DMPS treatment might be tolerated to correctly diagnose urine mercury concentration. Do not have anything to do with DMPS again. DMPS is too dangerous.

See Appendix III: http://www.sonic.net/~nexus/amalgam.html.

Use of Mercury Containing Restorations (Fillings) in Dentistry: Dr. Gordon J. Christensen: http://www.toothinfo.com/dht.htm

World Health Organization: http://www.who.ch

This is one of the best web pages on the Internet about the dental connection to chronic disease: http://www.biodent.com.au

The link between dental fillings and disease: www.vimy-dentistry.com/nhanesgraphs.htm

Root Canal Links

ALT, Inc.: solving problems dentistry, medicine and science: http://www.altcorp.com

Clinical Features of NICO: http://www.maxillofacialcenter.com/NICOclinical.html

Jaw Bone Infections, Causes and Cures: http://www.pnf.org/jaw_bone_infection.html

NICO Ultrasonic Imaging: http://www.maxillofacialcenter.com/NICOultrasound.html

Root Canal and Biocompatible Dentistry: http://www.zip.com.au/~rgammal/index.html

Root Canals and Cavitations: http://www.holisticmed.com/dental/root.html

Root Canals Pose Health Threat: An Interview with Dr. George Meinig: http://rheumatic.org/teeth.htm

Fluoride Links

AD Vision of Canada: http://www.cadvision.com/fluoride

Fluoridation/Fluoride Toxic Chemicals In Your Water: http://www.holisticmed.com/fluoride

IAOMT Risk Assessment For Ingested Fluoride: http://www.SaveTeeth.org

International Society for Fluoride Research: http://www.fluoride-journal.com

Stop Fluoridation USA: http://www.rvi.net/~fluoride

Why EPA's Headquarters Union of Scientists Opposes Fluoridation:

http://www.cadvision.com/fluoride/epa2.htm

Zero Waste America: http://www.zerowasteamerica.org/Fluoride.htm

Pro-Amalgam Link

American Dental Association (ADA): http://www.ada.org

In Vitro Treatment of a Neuroblastoma Cell Line with Low Concentrations of Thimerosal Results in Apoptosis and Altered Nucleotide Binding.

Specific Aim: to identify specific enzymes in the cell with emphasis on mitochondrial localization which are targets of Thimerosal toxicity.

We have previously reported that Hg is a potent inhibitor of a number of important nucleotide binding proteins in the human brain.[151,152] Treatment of human control brain homogenates with low (1-3 μM) concentrations of Hg in vitro induces aberrant protein-nucleotide in-

151 Pendergrass, J.C., and Haley, B.E. (1996) Inhibition of brain μtubulin-guanosine 5'-triposphate interactions by mercury: Similarity of observations in Alzheimer's disease. In: "Metal Ions in Biological Systems" (Sigel, H. and Sigel A. eds.) p 461-478. Marcel Dekker, Inc. New York.

152 Pendergrass, J.C. and Haley, B.E. (1995) "Mercury-EDTA complex specifically blocks brain b-tubulin-GTP interactions: similarity to observations in Alzheimer's disease." Status Quo and Perspectives of Amalgam and other dental materials (Friberg, L.T. and Schrauzer, G.N. eds.) p. 98-105. George Thieme Verlag, Stuttgart.

153 Duhr, E.F., Pendergrass J.C., Slevin, J.T., and Haley, B.E. (1993) HgEDTA complex inhibits GTP interactions with the E-site of brain b-tubulin. Toxicology and Applied Pharmacology 122, 273-280.

teractions characteristic of Alzheimer's disease (AD), a disease where brain Hg levels have been reported to be elevated.[153] Moreover, we have shown that two-week exposure of rats to elemental Hg vapor at levels present in the mouths of persons with high numbers of amalgam fillings results in the same aberrant protein-nucleotide interactions found in AD.[154] Recently our laboratory has found that Thimerosal is capable of inhibiting the activity of a number of critical mammalian nucleotide binding proteins (including but not limited to: creatine kinase, adenylate kinase, phosphoglycerate kinase, pryuvate kinase) in vitro at low (< 5 μM) levels, a fraction of what is actually included in many vaccines.[155] (Dr. Kelly Kiningham, Dr. Curt Pendergrass, President, ALT Inc., and Assistant Director, TEST Foundation, Lexington, KY).

The FASEB Journal.[156] 1998; 12:971-980.

Potential toxicity from exposure to Hg° from dental amalgam fillings is the subject of current public health debate in many countries. We evaluated potential central nervous system (CNS) toxicity associated with handling Hg-containing amalgam materials among dental personnel with very low-levels of Hg° exposure (i.e., Hg <4 ug/1 applying a neurobehavioral test battery to evaluate CNS functions in relation to both recent exposure and Hg body burden). New distinctions between subtle preclinical effects on symptoms, mood, motor function, and cognition were found associated with Hg body burden as compared with those associated with recent exposure. The pattern of

154 Pendergrass, J.C., and Haley, B.E., Vimy, M.J., Winfield, S.A., and Lorscheider, F.L (1997) Mercury vapor inhalation inhibits binding of GTP to tubulin in rat brain: Similarity to a molecular lesion in Alzheimer diseased brain. Neurotoxicology 18, 315-324.

155 Graduate Center for Toxicology, University of Kentucky, Lexington, KY, and Dr. Pendergrass, President, ALT Inc., and Assistant Director, TEST Foundation, Lexington, KY.

156 Federation of American Societies for Experimental Biology.

results, comparable to findings previously reported among subjects with urinary Hg >50 ug/1, presents convincing new evidence of adverse behavioral effects associated with low Hg° exposures within the range of that received by the general population.

Battelle Centers for Public Health Research and Evaluation, Seattle, WA 98105, USA

Department of Environmental Health, University of Washington, Seattle, WA 98195, USA

Department of Molecular and Cellular Biology, University of Arizona, Tucson, AZ 85721, USA

Echeverria, D., Aposhian, H. V., Woods, J. S., Heyer, N. J., Aposhian, M. M., Bittner, A. C., Jr., Mahurin, R. K. Neurobehavioral effects from exposure to dental amalgam Hg°: new distinctions between recent exposure and Hg body burden. FASEB .1: 12, 971-980 (1998)

Department of Psychiatry, University of Washington, Seattle, WA 98105, USA.

Toluene CASRN: 108-88-3

Hazardous Substances Data Bank

Toluene appears to produce reversible effects upon liver, renal, and nervous systems. The nervous system appears to be the most sensitive to the effects of toluene. High-level toluene exposures produced lack of coordination, ataxia, unconsciousness and, eventually, death. Lower-level acute exposures in man produce dizziness, exhilaration and confusion.

(Author) Toluene is an extremely toxic chemical that poisons the brain and central nervous system. Limited research suggests Toluene could cause short-term memory loss all by itself.

Appendix XIII

1: J Nucl Med 1992 Mar; 33(3):409-12

Nuclear medicine and acupuncture meridians message transmission.

De Vernejoul P, Albarede P. Darras JC.

2. Bull Acad Natl Med 1985 Oct;169(7):1071-5

[Study of acupuncture meridians using radioactive tracers]

[Article in French]

De Vernejoul P, Albarede P, Darras JC.

PMID: 3008958 [PubMed - indexed for MEDLINE]

3. Agressologie 1984 Nov; 25(10):1107-11

[Isotopic approach to the visualization of acupuncture meridians]

[Article in French]

de Verncjoul P, Darras JC, Beguin C, Gazalaa JB, Dqury G, Vernejoul J.

PMID: 6097132 [PubMed - indexed for MEDLINE]

Dr. Jerry Bouquot

The Maxillofacial Center for Education and Research
165 Scott Avenue, Suite 100, Morgantown, West Virginia, USA
(304) 292-4429 — bouquot@aol.com —fax: (304) 291-5649

Dr. Jerry Bouquot (pronounced Boko) received his D.D.S. and M.S. degrees from the University of Minnesota, with postdoctoral fellowships to the Mayo Clinic and the Royal Dental College in Copenhagen, Denmark as the recipient of a Career Development Award from the American Cancer Society. For almost two decades he was Professor and Chairman of the Department of Oral & Maxillofacial Pathology, West Virginia University. During that time, he received West Virginia University's highest teaching award and that University's highest award for service to the state.

He is the Director of Research for the Maxillofacial Center for Diagnostics and Research in Morgantown, West Virginia. He is also the Director of a large national biopsy service, Head & Neck Diagnostics of America. His federally (CLIA) certified lab receives tissue from 45 U.S. states and 7 other countries. He has been the Dental Director for the state of West Virginia, a Senior Visiting Scientist of the Mayo Clinic, a Special Advisor to the National Institutes of Health, and an Honorary Member of Dental Informatics of the University of Göteborg, in Sweden. He is a Consultant to Pittsburgh Children's Hospital, the New York Eye & Ear Infirmary, and the Clarksburg VA Hospital in West Virginia. He is a Professor of Dental Medicine at Capital University School of Integrated Medicine in Washington, D.C., an Adjunct Professor in the West Virginia University Schools of Dentistry and Medicine, a Fellow of the International College of Dentists, and a

Fellow of the Academy of Dentistry Internationale.

Dr. Bouquot has more than 180 published papers, abstracts and book chapters. His work has been translated into several languages, has been cited many hundreds of times in the literature, and has been used by state and national governments to determine oral health policy. He is co-author of the most popular textbook of Oral Pathology, has been a reviewer for more than 15 medical and dental journals, and is on the editorial boards of two international journals. He has presented more than 1,100 research and continuing education seminars and courses worldwide.

Dr. Bouquot has been President of the American Board of Oral & Maxillofacial Pathology and an Executive Councilor of the American Academy of Oral & Maxillofacial Pathology. He has been President of 3 regional dental societies, President five times of his state's American Cancer Society, and a member of the national Board of Directors of the American Cancer Society. As a member of the ACS national Research Committee he was among those responsible for reviewing and approving more than $90,000,000 in cancer research grants annually. He now serves on that organization's National Assembly, is on the Board of Trustees for the 5-state Mid-Atlantic Division of the ACS, and is President of an ACS region representing 25 counties of West Virginia and Maryland.

Jawbone Infection

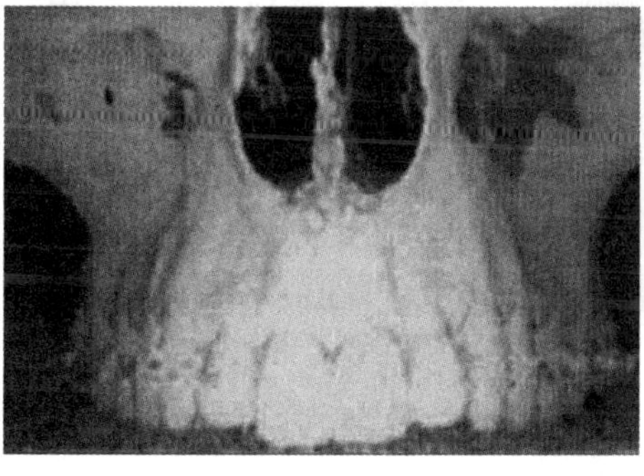

This image of the midface of a NICO patient shows perforation of the sinus walls, bilaterally.

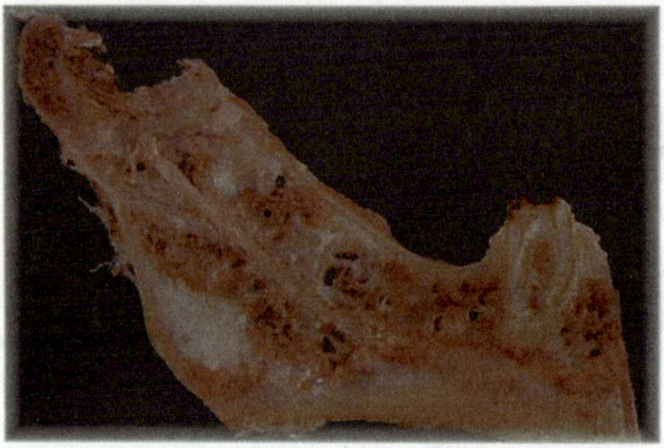

Massive ischemic damage to lower jaw, apparently from chemotherapy.

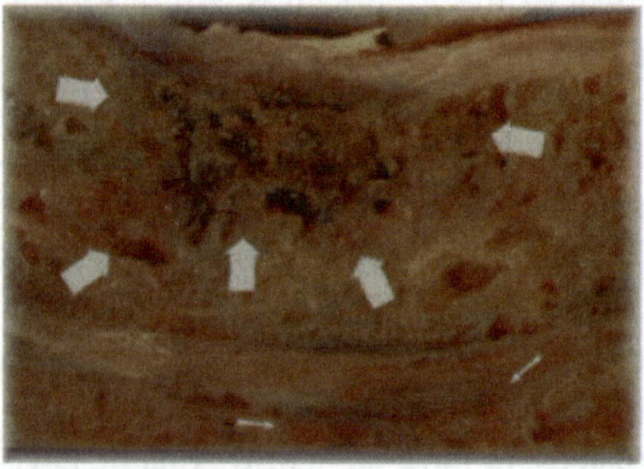

Maxillofacial Osteonecrosis (NICO).

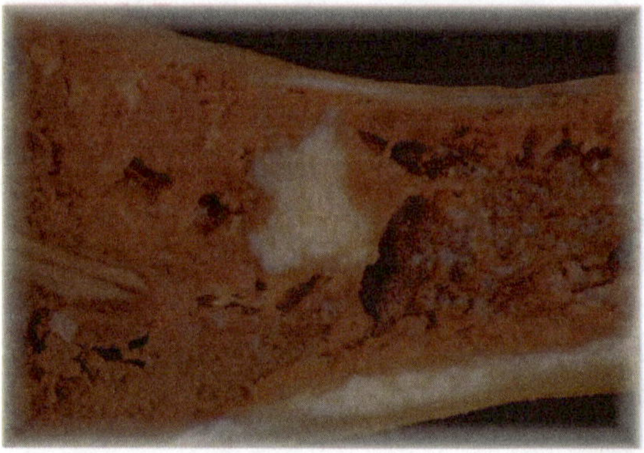

Large hollow space (above) in a severely ischemic mandible, with a generalized brown discoloration (degenerated fat and fibrosis) and large area of osteosclerosis (irregular white "bone island").

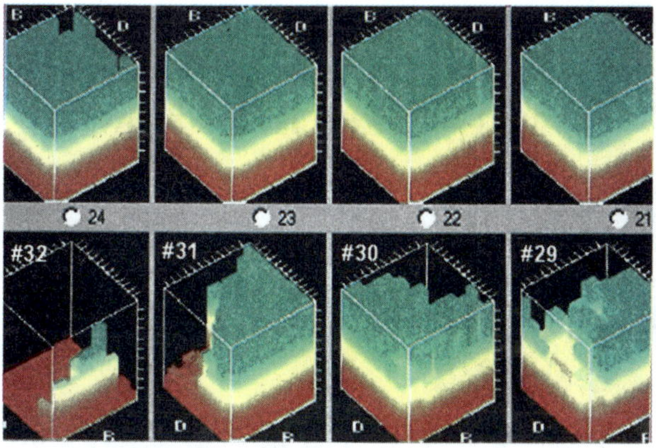

Cavitat Scan of Jawbone Infection.

Through-transmission ultrasonography cubes (3-dimensional graph; short, red/yellow columns= stopped sound)

Dr. Bouquot's most recent research:

93. Bouquot JE, LaMarche MG. Ischemic osteonecrosis under fixed partial denture pontics: radiographic and microscopic features in 38 patients with chronic pain. 2000 Yearbook of Dentistry. Year Book Med. Publ, Inc, Chicago, 2000. (abstract of publication #57).

94. Bouquot JE. The Oral Pathology Home Page. A public service website pertaining to all aspects of oral pathology and oral medicine. Opened June, 2000 at oralpath.com (receiving 10-20 hits daily).

95. Bouquot J, McMahon R The hollow tuberosity - clinicopathologic review of 1,057 biopsied cases. J Oral Pathol Med 2000; 29:345. (abstract). (abstract).

96. Bouquot J, Wrobleski G, Fenton S. The most common osteonecrosis? Prevalence of maxillofacial osteonecrosis (MFO). J Oral Pathol Med 2000; 29:345. (abstract).

97. Bouquot J, McMahon R. Bone marrow edema in maxillofacial osteonecrosis - clinicopathologic review of 2432 cases. Oral Surg Oral Med Oral Pathol Oral Radiol Endod 2000; 90:491. (abstract).

98. Bouquot J, Weiland L, Kurland L. A 58-year incidence of salivary neoplasms: striking increase for adenomas, decrease for adenocarcinomas. Oral Surg Oral Med Oral Pathol Oral Radiol Endod 2000; 90:491-492. (abstract).

99. Bouquot JE. Neuropathic pain in maxillofacial osteonecrosis. Proceedings of the 8th Salzburg Weekend Seminar, European Association for Cranio-Maxillofacial Surgery. Salzburg, Austria; October, 2000. (invited review).

100. Bouquot J, Adams W, Spolnik K, Deardorf K. Technetium-99m MDP (tech99) radioisotope bone scans & bone biopsies in 56 patients with chronic facial pain. Oral Surg Oral Med Oral Pathol Oral Radiol Endod 2001; 92:543. (abstract).

101.Bouquot J, Martin W, Wrobleski G. Computer-based thru-transmission sonography (CTS) imaging of ischemic osteonecrosis of the jaws - a preliminary investigation of 6 cadaver jaws and 15 pain patients. Oral Surg Oral Med Oral Pathol Oral Radiol Endod 2001; 92:550. (abstract).

102. Fisher MA, Bouquot JE. Assessment of risk factors for oral leukoplakia. Proceedings, National Oral Health Conference, Danvers, Massachusetts; April, 2002. (abstract).

103. Bouquot JE, Margolis M, Shankland WE. Through-transmission sonography (TTS) - new technology for the evaluation of jawbone density and dessication. Correlation with histopathology of 285 scanned alveolar sites. Proceedings of annual meeting, American Academy of Oral & Maxillofacial Pathology, New Orleans, Louisiana; April, 2002. (tentative).

104. Bouquot JE, Shankland WE, Margolis M. Through-transmission sonography (TTS) - new technology for evaluation of bone density and dessication. Comparison with radiology of 170 biopsied alveolar sites of osteoporotic and ischemic damage. Proceedings of annual meeting, American Academy of Oral & Maxillofacial Pathology, New Orleans, Louisiana; April, 2002. (tentative).

105. Bouquot JE, Rohrer M, McMahon RE, Boc T. Focal osteoporotic marrow defect (FOMD) - literature review and report of 596 new cases. Proceedings of annual meeting, American Academy of Oral & Maxillofacial Pathology, New Orleans, Louisiana; April, 2002. (tentative).

106. Bouquot JE, Gnepp DR. Erythroplakia and carcinoma in situ - head and neck lesions revisited. Proceedings of annual meeting, American Academy of Oral Medicine, Ft. Lauderdale, Florida; April, 2002. (tentative).

107. Bouquot JE, Fisher M, Young S. Human papillomavirus types 16/18 in 355 oral leukoplakias. Bouquot J, Fisher M, Young S, Proceedings of annual meeting, American Academy of Oral Medicine, Ft. Lauderdale, Florida; April, 2002. (tentative).

For further information and research papers about jawbone infection go to Dr. Bouquot's Webpage at http://www.maxillofacialcenter.com. If you haven't already, read Chapter II in Section I of this book.

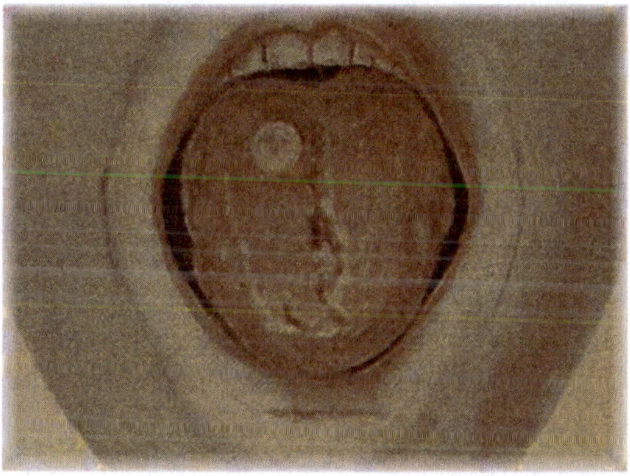

This person needs to clean his or her tongue with a tablespoon.

I have seen thousands of split tongues of people who have mercury poisoning, schizophrenia, Alzheimer's disease, cancer and dozens of other medical problems. One gentleman who was being sent home to die from cancer had so many holes in his tongue it looked as if his tongue had been repeatedly hit by the tines of a steel garden rake. I told the Mexican director of the hospital what to do and two years later a friend called to tell me that my information caused every cancer clinic in Mexico to remove the patient's mercury fillings, first. The identical approach to treatment is used by the Paracelsus Clinic at Lüstmuhle, Switzerland.

In Chapter I, I mentioned a schizophrenic mental patient who was hospitalized at Washington's Eastern and Western State Hospitals for 35 years. His tongue was split right down the middle. There was barely a quarter of an inch of tissue left before two or two and one half inches of his tongue would have split in two. I told the patient's nurse and psychiatrist what to do and as far as his mental health was concerned, he could have been released within three months, but there were legal issues that needed to be resolved. It took awhile longer.

If I do not take my vitamins and minerals every day, my tongue begins to split. Mercury poisoning shuts off HCl (stomach acid) causing acute malnutrition.

Root Canal Treatment: Is there a cover-up?

By Wesley E. Shankland, II, D.D.S., M.S., Ph.D.

For the past 50 years, dentists have saved millions of teeth by performing endodontic therapy, or root canals. Dental students and residents in Endodontics (the speciality in dentistry devoted to the diagnosis and treatment of diseases inside teeth) have been taught to perform various procedures to save injured, dead, and dying teeth. These procedures were taught purely to help the public, with absolutely no other reason. The dental profession succeeded in teaching the value of saving teeth. However, today, there has been some revealing research which may require the dental profession to reconsider conventional ideas about endodontically treated teeth.

Today, there are many reputable doctors (dentists, physicians, and PhDs) who are concerned about endodontic therapy and possbile systemic effects on other organs and tissues in the body. It may even astound most dentists that the organisms which may be present in dead teeth may be impossible to irradicate no matter how well the root canal procedure is performed! These organisms are not actually in the canal portion of the tooth, but in the tiny microscopic tubules which comprise the dentin (the material below the enamel which is more organic than enamel) of the tooth. Herein lies the scientific question: does it matter that these organisms remain viable even after endodontic therapy? Researchers on both sides of this heated issue agree that these organisms do stay alive after root canal procedures, but they can't agree whether this is important or not.

Dr. Weston Price, the noted and honored dental researcher of the early part of this century, headed a team of America's finest scientific researchers, numbering 60 doctors. Their research was conducted under the auspices of the American Dental Association (ADA). From their 25 years of study, this research team published 25 scientific papers dealing with the effects of dead or endodontically treated teeth producing other diseases and disorders in remote areas of the body.

The research was not only accepted by the scientific community, but served to form an important concept in medicine which is even taught today: the focal theory of infection. Anyone who has a prosthetic joint replacement or a mitral value prolapse will immediately understand this concept, as they cannot undergo any dental procedure without first being treated with certain antibiotics to stop the spread of bacteria from the mouth to remote areas of the body which may produce a fatal infection.

Since the advent of antibiotics, dentists and physicians have been taught that the focal theory of infection is erroneous and has no scientific basis. Further, they are taught that there is no modern evidence that endodontically treated teeth are the source of focal infections. However, again, recall that patients with joint replacements and certain heart conditions must take antibiotics before and after any dental procedures. Why? Because the bacteria which live in the mouth enter the blood stream because of the dental procedures and travel to the heart and joints, thus possibily causing severe and often fatal diseases. Now, think about what you've just read: how can any dentist or physician claim that the focal theory of infection has no scientific validity when dentists are required to premedicate their patients to avoid producing a distant or focal infection?

Who's Guarding the Hen House?

I would have preferred to present this information to the public and let them draw their own conclusions, but someone has to lay it on the line, because the Washington State Dental Board's past-record of serving the public interest reeks of chicanery and evasion of responsibility.

Mercury amalgam dental fillings poison every cell in the body. Endodontists leave infected root canals in our jawbones that discharge toxins into our blood stream, which in time, when our immune system cannot hold back the tide any longer, cause horrific chronic diseases.

(1) Most photographs of infected jawbone (pages 258-260) originate from cadavers. (2) Almost everyone has jawbone infection caused by sloppy dental housekeeping. (3)Neither mainstream ADA dentists nor the Washington State Dental Board are going to admit they have misled the public about these issues.

Else, why would the Washington State Dental Board force dentists to sign consent decrees not to do oral surgery to clean up cavitations or face the loss of their license? If that is not cover-up, what is? It appears the dental board is trying to muffle the very specialists who have the experience to teach our university students the procedures that will drag the dental community into the 21st Century. Apparently, the reputations of the ADA and AAE, our dental schools and the income they generate are more important than the dental patient's health if it exposes the dental communities' incompetence to the public.

The American Dental Association and the American Association of Endodontists act like trade guilds whose interests are in their members, not us. They should be paying the Washington State Dental Board's salary, not taxpayers. The best solution is to fire the whole dental board and replace them with dentists and two private citizens, hopefully one would be a newspaper reporter, whose foremost interest is the dental patient's health.

Statement by Congresswoman Diane Watson

Mercury in Dental Filling Disclosure and Prohibition Act

November 5, 2001

In times like these, there are toxins that we don't know about - how to control them, their source and their impact. But there are toxins that we DO know about - toxins that we know do not belong in our bodies, toxins that we can do something about. My bill addresses that very problem.

Mercury is an acute neurotoxin. It is the most toxic non-radioactive element and the most volatile heavy metal. In recent years, it has been, or is being removed from all health care uses, save one. Antibiotics have replaced oral doses of Mercury. The disinfectant Mercurochrome is banned. Recently, the Centers for Disease Control ordered Mercury preservatives removed from childhood vaccines. Mercury preservatives are no long used in contact lens solutions. This year, legislatures in California and several other states banned Mercury thermometers. When Governor Gray Davis signed bills addressing Mercury in thermometers and in dental fillings, he said, "Mercury is a persistent and toxic pollutant that bioaccumulates in the environment." In recent years, the American Public Health Association, the California Medical Association and Health Care Without Harm have all called for the elimination of putting any Mercury in the human body.

Today, I am announcing legislation to disclose and phase-out the last major use of Mercury in the human body. The fillings that organized dentistry wrongly calls "silver" are mainly Mercury, not "silver."

Mercury is the major ingredient in each filling, about one-half gram per. In the words of Professor Boyd Haley of the University of Kentucky, that is a "colossal" amount of Mercury in scientific terms - as much, in fact, as is in a thermometer. A teenager with six fillings has six Mercury thermometers worth of Mercury in his or her mouth.

The Mercury in the fillings is volatile, such that - as all authorities concede - poisonous vapors are constantly being emitted from the fillings, more so when one chews or passes hot liquid over the teethe. The Agency for Toxic Substances & Disease Registry of the United States Public Health Service reports that those poisonous vapors go first to the brain and kidneys. For the developing brain - and by that I mean a child's brain - a major health risk exists.

It is in fact children who are at greatest risk from these fillings. The government of Canada recommended back in 1996 that dentists not place fillings in the mouths of children or pregnant women. (The 1999 report on Mercury by the Agency for Toxic Substances & Disease Registry says Mercury passes through the placenta into the developing child's brain.) In 1997, a major manufacturer of dental amalgam, Dentsply, said that amalgam is CONTRAINDICATED (translation DO NOT USE) for children and pregnant women, as well as for those with braces, Mercury hypersensitivities, or kidney problems. Another manufacturer, Vivadent, added a contraindication for nursing mothers. (The 1999 government report says the Mercury goes through the mother's breast milk into the baby.)

Why don't consumers already know this? The answer is a disappointing one. Organized dentistry is extremely divided on this issue. My bill, in fact is supported by the American Academy of Biological Dentistry. But the American Dental Association tells the public that the fillings are safe. The ADA does not tell the public that it accepts payments from the amalgam manufacturers while it pronounces their product safe. I wish to note that the American Medical Association has a policy prohibiting the organization from taking money for product endorsements. The ADA, by contrast, accepts money from the manufacturers of the products it endorses which certainly hurts its credibility in my mind.

The public does not know about the presence of Mercury and its risks for two reasons. First, the fillings are falsely called "silver." This term is deceptive, because there is much more Mercury than silver in the product. It's time to call it what it is and quit hiding the large presence of Mercury.

Second, the ADA has a rule that gags dentists from talking about the risks of Mercury amalgam, a rule that some dental boards enforce against dentists who call for the elimination of Mercury in dental fillings. I understand that rule is being challenged by dentists in federal court in Maryland based on the First Amendment.

Developments in this area have been quite encouraging this year in my state. In 1992, as a state Senator, I wrote a law that required the Dental Board of California to write a "Fact Sheet" about the risks and efficacies of dental fillings. My goal was to ensure the public could make informed choices about Mercury dental amalgam. But the Dental Board continued to ignore the law and, in recent years, defy the Davis Administration's insistence that it comply with this law. After an impasse, including the Board refusing to show up for a hearing in Los Angeles on this issue, the Legislature stepped in and shut down the Board. I am told that never before has the California Legislature shut down a board before its Sunset date expired. In January, a new Dental Board will come into existence.

A major environmental issue exists here. When removed from a patient's mouth, Mercury amalgam is a hazardous waste, and it is often improperly disposed of. The more Mercury that goes into people's teeth, the more of it that will end up in our water supply. I am delighted, therefore, that San Francisco-based Clean Water Action is supporting my bill, and I look forward to other environmental groups joining us in this effort.

The occupational risk is significant. Dental employees are constantly exposed to the vapors. Women in dental offices have lower fecundity (pregnancy) rates, more miscarriages, and more problem births. Mercury exposure is the likely reason. Dentists have the highest suicide rate of any profession; depression leading to suicide is consistent with a diagnosis of Mercury toxicity.

Mercury amalgam is dangerous before it is put in the mouth - any dental journal will tell you that - and it is considered hazardous waste after it has been removed. Who can conclusively say it's safe in between when it is in our bodies?

A major social justice, or environment justice, issue exists here. While the public lacks informed choice, low- and moderate-income people have it worse: they have no choice at all. For families on Medi-Cal, the children get Mercury - or nothing. It is outrageous that low-income Americans are forced to have such a toxic material put in their mouths. I understand that the Rhode Island legislature adopted a law this year to provide choice in insurance plans, and that the state of Maine permits Medicaid children to get alternatives to amalgam - so, yes, we can do it differently.

Mercury, and all other poisons in the body, hurt the body's immune system - its ability to withstand diseases and biologically harmful agents. If at any time in our nations history we need strong immune systems, it is now. The stronger our bodies, the more able we are to fend off biological agents that have so tragically been placed in our midst.

My bill will protect children, pregnant women, and nursing mothers immediately - regardless of their income. Henceforth, amalgam will bear warnings that they not be placed in these most vulnerable people. And there will be health warnings for all consumers of amalgam, also immediately. Then, there is a five-year phase out of Mercury amalgam. That will give dentistry plenty of time to shift to alternatives that exist in today's market - resin, porcelain, and gold - or to develop new materials.

Dentistry says amalgam is fine because it has been in ;use for 150 years. This statement makes no scientific sense. We have abandoned other remnants of pre-Civil War medicine, and we have abandoned all other uses of Mercury. It is no longer a question of if, but when. Mercury dental fillings will be history. I say five more years is time enough.

Congresswoman Diane Watson

5100 Goldleaf Circle, Suite 208

Los Angeles, CA 90056

Washington DC 20515

Statement by Congressman Dan Burton

Chairman of the Committee for Government Reform

Mercury in Dental Amalgams and Vaccines: An Examination of the Science

November 14, 2002

Over the last three years, the Government Reform Committee has looked at health and safety issues related to Mercury-containing products.

In July 2000, we held a hearing titled, "Mercury in Medicine - Are we Taking Unnecessary Risks?" We focused on why mercury is put into vaccines that are given to children. We received a report during that hearing that indicated that the symptoms of mercury toxicity are similar to the symptoms of autism.

That was followed-up by a hearing on April 18, 2002, entitled, "The Autism Epidemic - Is the NIH and CDC Response Adequate?"

We have conducted numerous hearings on the Vaccine Injury Compensation Program. I am pleased that Dr. Dave Weldon and our Ranking Minority Member, Congressman Waxman joined me in co-sponsoring legislation to improve the Compensation Program. I believe through our oversight activities that we have made it absolutely clear to the Department of Justice and the Department of Health and Human Services that the intent of Congress was and remains that the National Vaccine Injury Compensation Program should be a no-fault compensation program, not a contentious tort system. I really regret that we haven't been able to get this bill passed, because it would really help people.

Today's hearing will focus primarily on the science regarding mercury-containing dental amalgams.

Early on in our investigation, I was accused of being "anti-vaccine."

Now that we are examining the science behind the use of mercury in dental amalgams, I suppose I'll be characterized as anti-dentistry. Neither charge could be further from the truth!

Immunizations have been portrayed as one of the greatest advances in public health during the past century, second only to clean water and improved hygiene. I think that's true-although we need to make sure vaccines are as safe as possible. Dentistry is a noble profession that has contributed to Americans' overall health and quality of life. While immunizations may offer great benefit, they also carry risks. And while dentistry offers great benefit, the continued use of a toxic substance such as mercury needs examination.

Mercury is mercury, whether it is methyl or ethyl, organic or inorganic. There is no one in this room or in all of science who can say with any level or credibility that any form of mercury is safe. While many people have absolutely no problem from being injected with thimerosal-containing vaccines; and while mercury-containing dental amalgams have been used for over 150 years, we have a responsibility to protect those who are pregnant women, infants and young children, those with autoimmune dysfunction, and the elderly.

And with dental amalgams, I'm also talking about economically disadvantaged people of all ages who depend upon Medicaid for dental care. They either get fillings with mercury, or no fillings at all.

Are we giving them short-term relief by helping pay for their dental work, only to set them up for disaster - for long-term problems down the road?

The simple fact is that Mercury is one of the most toxic minerals on earth, second only to radioactive materials.

The fillings that typically are called "Silver" fillings because of their color probably should be called mercury fillings. They consist of 50% or more of mercury. When the mercury is mixed with an alloy of powdered metals, it becomes Dental Amalgam.

For many years dental schools taught that when the amalgam hardens it becomes inert. They taught that there was no further risk from the mercury.

However, from research, we now know that mercury vapor continues to leech from amalgams for as long as it remains in the mouth. The fumes are inhaled into the human body and minute particles chip off and are ingested into the stomach as fillings wear.

This has important health implications, since mercury has a long half-life and has the potential for doing significant damage to the kidneys and brain. For reasons that are not well understood, some individuals seem to hold on to the mercury absorbed by their body, leaving them at risk for neurological or renal damage.

In 1999 the U.S. Agency for Toxic Substances and Disease Registry, published the Toxicological Profile in Mercury (Update). This report stated that poisonous mercury vapors are constantly emitted from amalgam, that these vapors go first to the brain, and that children are most at risk because their brains are still developing. The report further states that the mercury crosses the placenta to the developing fetus, and that it is transmitted through a mother's milk to the infant.

The Food and Drug Administration has taken what appears to be a bipolar approach to protecting the public from mercury. While denying that thimerosal in vaccines or mercury in dental amalgams poses any health risk, it has taken a stand against mercury in other products:

- The FDA has repeatedly issued strong warnings cautioning the pub lic, and in particular pregnant women and young children to re strict their consumption of tuna and other fish that is known to contain mercury.

- The FDA has determined that mercury compounds used as active ingredients in over-the-counter drug products were not "generally recognized as safe."

- They also have not approved any mercury-containing compounds as food additives.

- The FDA also states, "Lead, cadmium, and mercury are examples of elements that are toxic when present at relatively low levels.

I've asked before, and I'll ask again. How is it that mercury is not safe for food additives and over-the-counter drugs, but it is safe in our vaccines and in our dental fillings?

There are alternatives to mercury-containing amalgams. Shouldn't we exercise an abundance of caution and hasten the use of those alternatives?

Before I conclude, I want to commend Congresswoman Diane Watson of California for her initiative in sponsoring H.R. 4163, The Mercury in Dental Filling Disclosure and Prohibition Act.

As I've already stated, the federal government must exercise special care for vulnerable population groups. Physical and in particular neurological damage from mercury is an issue that crosses all boundaries - geographic, economic, ethnic, and religious, age, and gender - all boundaries!

It is said that you can't stop an idea whose time has come. Hasn't the time come to stop exposing people to mercury through medical interventions?

Congressman Dan Burton

2185 Rayburn HOB

Washington, DC 20515